W9-BNT-139

KEYS TO
LIVING WITH
HEARING LOSS

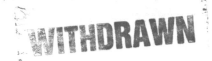

WITHDRAWN

KEYS TO
LIVING WITH
HEARING LOSS

Marcia B. Dugan

SCHAUMBURG TOWNSHIP DISTRICT LIBRARY
32 WEST LIBRARY LANE
SCHAUMBURG, ILLINOIS 60194

362.42
5/97 oub

3 1257 01119 3801

This book is dedicated to the millions of people who have accepted their hearing loss and educated themselves to live with it successfully, and to the many others who, after reading this book, take steps to help themselves live better with hearing loss.

© Copyright 1997 by Barron's Educational Series, Inc.

All rights reserved.
No part of this book may be reproduced in any form,
by photostat, microfilm, xerography, or any other means, or incorpo-
rated into any information retrieval system, electronic or mechanical,
without the written permission of the copyright owner.

All inquiries should be addressed to:
Barron's Educational Series, Inc.
250 Wireless Boulevard
Hauppauge, NY 11788

Library of Congress Catalog Card Number 96-54037

International Standard Book Number 0-7641-0017-3

Library of Congress Cataloging-in-Publication Data
Dugan, Marcia B.
    Keys to living with hearing loss / Marcia B. Dugan.
        p.   cm. — (Barron's keys to retirement planning)
    Includes bibliographical references and index.
    ISBN 0-7641-0017-3
    1. Aged, Deaf—Psychology. 2. Aged, Deaf—Means of communication.
    3. Hearing impaired—Rehabilitation. 4. Adjustment (Psychology) in old age.
    I. Title. II. Series.
    HV2393.D85   1997
    362.4'2'0846—dc21   96-54037
                                                     CIP

PRINTED IN THE UNITED STATES OF AMERICA

987654321

CONTENTS

FOREWORD

When people suspect that they have a hearing loss, their initial response is often to pretend that they don't have a problem or to assume that nothing can help them. Yet, losing our hearing requires us to modify the way we communicate and therefore can affect every element of our lives because we communicate in countless ways—not just when we are speaking face to face or on the telephone.

Hearing loss affects people of all ages, but it is more common as we get older. At least one third of people over age 65 have some level of hearing loss. How discouraging it can be to suddenly realize that we cannot communicate as we have always done! But having a hearing loss doesn't mean that we must stop doing the things we have enjoyed all our lives.

As a hard of hearing person who began losing my hearing in my late twenties, I experienced firsthand both the emotional and practical adjustments that people must make if they wish to remain a part of the mainstream. When I began searching for tools to help me, a book like this—written by someone who had personally experienced the complexities of hearing loss—was not in print. Nor did I have the benefit of information and support provided by Self Help for Hard of Hearing People, Inc. (SHHH).

Marcia Dugan has been actively involved in SHHH for more than a decade, and her development of this book reflects her own experiences with hearing loss as well as those of the thousands of people who have communicated with SHHH during our 18 years of existence. The 41 keys presented in this book distill into a very short space the philosophy on which we were founded and the reason we continue to exist: People can help themselves live better with hearing loss if they have the information they need to take action and be in control of their lives.

It is with enormous pleasure and pride that we can now share what our members have taught us with people everywhere.

Donna L. Sorkin
Executive Director
Self Help for Hard of Hearing People, Inc.
7910 Woodmont Avenue, Suite 1200
Bethesda, Maryland 20814

PREFACE

It is difficult for people who do not have a hearing loss to understand what a hard of hearing person experiences. Many people who hear well think that all you have to do is turn up the volume and ask others to speak louder.

The real problem with hearing loss, however, is that it creates a barrier to communication. It can prevent a person from having normal conversations with family and friends, in the workplace, and on the telephone; enjoying TV, the movies, theater, and music; and participating in public activities, meetings, and group assemblies.

Older Americans don't have to give up the lifestyle they enjoy if they acknowledge their hearing loss, seek information, and learn how they can help themselves; however, they often delay in learning to live with their hearing loss. Many retire early because of the stresses of working in a job setting with no accommodations for their disability. Others have health conditions that take precedence over doing something about their hearing loss. It is also sad that older people with hearing loss often are targeted by mail order hearing aid sales and other marketing schemes at a time when many live on limited or fixed income.

The information in this compilation of short keys reflects my own experience with hearing loss and the knowledge I acquired while finding out what to do about it in order to remain in the mainstream. It was written to help you learn to live with your hearing loss. Living with a hearing loss does not mean giving in to it; many communication strategies and assistive devices are available to ease the difficulties of understanding speech. You will find out that a great deal can be done to improve communication, even though your hearing loss cannot be changed.

Confucius said, "The essence of knowledge is, having it, to use it." I hope that readers of this book will use the knowledge gained from reading it to take the steps needed to live better with hearing loss.

Acknowledgments

It is with a special measure of gratitude that I thank Barron's for its interest in publishing a book on hearing loss as part of the Retirement Planning Series. As a strong believer that many older Americans have the potential to remain active and independent well into their later years, I am pleased to have the opportunity to provide information that can help those with hearing loss to do just that.

The information in the book was gleaned from a broad spectrum of resources: products, promotional materials, and publications, as well as from the experiences of many SHHH members who shared strategies for dealing with situations that often challenge people with hearing loss.

I am especially indebted to a number of people who through their expertise have made this book possible: SHHH national staff members Donna Sorkin, Brenda Battat, and Barbara Harris for helping me develop the concept, reviewing the keys, and offering suggestions; members of the SHHH Rochester Chapter, whose sharing of personal experiences with hearing loss provided insight and information for the experiential keys; the many contributors to *Hearing Loss: The Journal of Self Help for Hard of Hearing People*, whose articles provided background information; Linda Bement, M.S., CCC-A., Diane Castle, Ph.D., John Niparko, M.D., and Mark Ross, Ph.D., for their audiological and medical expertise; Julie Olson, former president of SHHH, for information regarding psychosocial effects of hearing loss; the writers on my former staff at the National Technical Institute for the Deaf, who wrote many of the brochures and *NTID Focus* articles from which I drew information and whose writing skills educated me; and a very special thank you to Susan Cergol, writer-editor *sin par*, whose suggestions while reviewing the final product permitted me to make it a clearer, better book.

Marcia B. Dugan

1

HEARING LOSS: THE EARLY SIGNS

It may be difficult to remember the first time you realized that you couldn't hear as well as you once did. Most hearing loss occurs gradually, so you may not have noticed that it was happening. You could hear some people; you had difficulty hearing others. You could hear in some situations; in other situations, you had a problem hearing. These mixed signals are confusing and often prevent people from acknowledging a hearing loss. For this reason, it often is a friend or family member who notices that a person is losing their hearing. Below are some of the warning signs of early hearing loss:

- You hear but cannot understand.
- You ask people to repeat what they said or respond inappropriately to questions.
- You have difficulty understanding in restaurants, the car, and other noisy environments where several people are talking at the same time.
- You have difficulty hearing at the movies or in the theater.
- You have difficulty understanding in group or social situations.
- You cannot understand your grandchildren or other young children.
- You hear better in one ear than in the other when you are on the telephone.
- You have dizziness, pain, or ringing in your ears.
- You turn the television and radio volume louder than other people like.

1

- You have difficulty understanding speech if you can't see the speaker's face.
- You turn your head to one side to hear what is said.

In addition to observing the above signs, your family may notice the following:
- You have a blank expression on your face.
- You speak too loudly or too softly.
- You can't understand what is being said when someone speaks to you from another room.
- You avoid social situations.
- You tune out or fall asleep at group gatherings.

Denial
The average delay between the onset of hearing loss and seeking a professional diagnosis is five to seven years. One reason for this delay is not noticing the change in hearing in the early stages of acquired hearing loss. A more prevalent reason is failure to admit there is a problem or avoidance or denial of the problem. If you are in the denial stage, you may try to hide the loss because you may perceive it as a sign of aging or carrying the stigma of a disability. You also may hide your hearing loss by not participating in conversations, by smiling when everyone else is doing so, and by bluffing in other ways. Denial is exacerbated by the fact that in some situations you can hear and in others you cannot, so you waver between acceptance and denial of the need for a hearing test. The hearing loss is often obvious to your family members and friends; however, if you are like most hard of hearing people, at first you may blame your problem on others.

It Doesn't Hurt
Since hearing loss is usually free of physical pain, people who are hard of hearing tend to put off dealing with it, especially if they are also experiencing other physical

problems such as arthritis and heart disease. Although physically painless, hearing loss can cause you emotional pain since it makes you feel socially inept, isolated, embarrassed, even depressed. Poor hearing disrupts communication and can lead to unhappiness. It also can cause pain for your family and friends who may become frustrated and angry when trying to communicate (see Key 4).

Getting Help: Make It a Priority

If listening situations are causing you to strain, tune out, or feel fatigued and irritable, it may be time to admit you have a hearing loss. If so, this is the time to see a hearing health care specialist to determine what the problem is. Some hearing losses may be medically or surgically correctable; most can be helped by wearing a hearing aid. Much information is available when you decide that doing something about your hearing loss is your top priority.

Hearing your family and friends is vital to remaining happy, healthy, and in control of your life. Good communication with family and friends is especially important for older people. You owe it to yourself to have the best quality of life possible.

2

WHAT IS HEARING LOSS?

Hearing loss often occurs gradually, and you may not be aware that you have not been hearing as well as you once did. You may find you hear well in some situations and wonder why it is difficult for you to understand in others. Your family, friends, and co-workers may often have to repeat themselves so that you can understand them.

Unlike other disabilities, hearing loss is invisible. There are no wheelchairs, leg braces, or red-tipped canes to indicate that a person has a hearing loss. Yet, hearing loss is the most prevalent, least recognized, and least understood physical disability. *One of every ten people has a hearing loss.* And although not normal at any age, hearing loss is more common among older adults than in the general population. At age 65, one in every three persons has some degree of hearing loss, and the incidence is even higher among those of more advanced years.

Although hearing loss will require some changes, by acknowledging it and with help from professionals and technology—as well as self help—you can enjoy an independent and relaxed lifestyle. Like many others, you will discover new ways to adapt in order to fully participate in the world around you.

Remember: The real problem with a hearing loss is not the loss itself, but the barrier to communication it creates and the stress you may experience if you do not address it.

Degrees of Hearing Loss

Just as people have varying degrees of visual problems, individual hearing losses also are different and range from mild to profound (see Figure 1). The degree of hearing loss is measured in decibels (dB).

4

- If you have a *mild* hearing loss (26–45 dB), you may have difficulty hearing and understanding someone who is speaking from a distance or who has a soft voice. You also may have difficulty understanding conversations in noisy backgrounds.
- If your hearing loss is in the *moderate* range (46–65 dB), you will have difficulty understanding conversation in quiet backgrounds as well.
- If your hearing loss is *severe* (66–90 dB), you will have difficulty understanding conversations in all situations.
- If you have a *profound* hearing loss (greater than 90 dB), you may not even hear loud speech or environmental sounds.

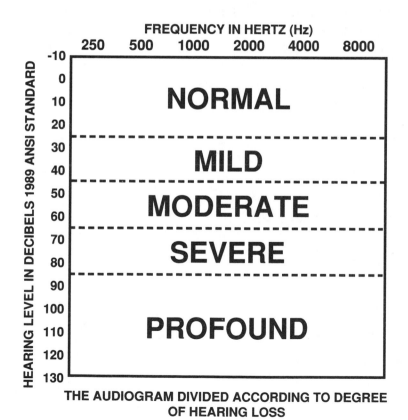

Figure 1 Degrees of Hearing Loss.

But volume is only part of the problem; sounds can also seem distorted. In other words, you can hear, but you cannot understand. This is because hearing loss has two parts: loudness and clarity.

Loudness. A person with a loudness problem usually will find it much easier to understand speech if sounds are made loud enough; some sounds, however, may never be loud enough to be heard.

Clarity. The person with a clarity problem finds sounds are unclear or cannot be understood at all even when amplified. Most hard of hearing people experience problems with both loudness and clarity.

Frequency. Frequency (pitch), which is important for understanding speech, is measured in hertz (Hz). You may have trouble hearing consonants like *s*, *f*, and *th*, but can still hear low-frequency sounds such as *ah*, *oo*, and *m*. This is because hearing loss for older people is usually greater in the high frequencies.

3

MYTHS ABOUT HEARING LOSS: FACT AND FICTION

Once you have acknowledged your hearing loss and decided to do something about it, you will receive advice—solicited and unsolicited—from family and friends, and even medical personnel.

Some of this advice and information is accurate, but a large amount of misinformation has been circulated over the years. Listed below are some incorrect statements and the corrected information to help you understand your hearing loss.

Myth: A mild hearing loss is nothing to be concerned about.

Truth: Although you may think that you are not missing important information and seem to be managing, you may not realize that your family and friends are frustrated and that you have begun to feel left out. Not only should you be concerned about your hearing loss, you should do something about it.

Myth: You will be the first person to notice that you have a hearing loss.

Truth: Because hearing loss often occurs gradually, you may not notice it at first. Family members and co-workers often are the first to notice that you need to have questions repeated or that the television is too loud.

Myth: Your hearing loss is normal for your age.

Truth: Hearing loss is not normal at any age; however, hearing loss is more prevalent among older adults than in the general population. Currently, approximately one third of the population older than 65 has some degree of hearing loss.

Myth: You have a sensorineural hearing loss (nerve deafness) and there is nothing you can do about it.

Truth: Most hearing losses can be helped with amplification and assistive listening devices. A majority of people with nerve deafness hear better by wearing hearing aids. This form of hearing loss is not correctable with surgery. Conductive hearing loss, however, is often correctable medically or surgically.

Myth: You would understand people if you listened more carefully.

Truth: Although paying attention, watching the speaker's lips, and observing body language can help you understand the message, no amount of careful listening can make you understand what you can't hear clearly. If you have a hearing loss, you need to acknowledge it and see a trained hearing health care professional for an evaluation to determine if you would benefit from a hearing aid.

Myth: Your hearing loss is not bad enough for a hearing aid.

Truth: Everyone's hearing loss is different. Some hard of hearing people hear well on the telephone; others have difficulty. Some have no problem in a quiet one-on-one situation but have difficulty in a noisy or group setting. You must determine the degree of difficulty you are having, and together with a trained hearing health care professional, determine your need for a hearing aid.

Myth: A hearing aid will correct your hearing.

Truth: A hearing aid may be helpful, but it is not a cure for hearing loss. Hearing aids will not restore hearing loss to normal. If your hearing loss can be helped with a hearing aid, then an appropriately prescribed and fitted hearing aid should make your hearing and understanding abilities better, and in turn, improve your quality of life.

Myth: A hearing aid will damage your hearing.

Truth: A hearing aid will *not* damage your hearing.

Myth: Your hearing loss is not bad enough for two hearing aids.

Truth: We normally hear with two ears; therefore, most people with hearing loss in both ears can understand better with two aids than with one.

Myth: Behind-the-ear hearing aids are old fashioned; you will do much better with the newer in-the-ear hearing aids.

Truth: Behind-the-ear hearing aids are as "state of the art" as in-the-ear hearing aids. Some include features not found in the smaller hearing aids, and a particular feature may be important for you. You should work closely with your hearing health care provider to ensure that the aid you get is appropriate for your particular needs. Function, not appearance, is the crucial consideration.

Myth: You should have your hearing tested in your own home where you spend most of your time.

Truth: The hearing test should be conducted in a soundproof room in order to provide the most accurate results. The information gleaned from the test is used to select the most appropriate hearing aid for your individual hearing loss. Only individuals confined to a bed for health reasons should have hearing tests in other sites such as their home.

Myth: You can save a lot of money buying a hearing aid through the mail.

Truth: When you buy a hearing aid, you not only are buying a piece of equipment, you are buying the service of a hearing health care provider in your locality. Unlike eyeglasses, hearing aids require a longer period of adjustment and often modifications that can only be made by trained personnel. The wrong hearing aid, or one that is not fitted properly, can be worse than no hearing aid at all.

Myth: Your hearing loss will not change in the future.

Truth: No one can predict the future. Your hearing loss may remain stable for the rest of your life, or it may change slowly and progressively or suddenly and dramatically.

Myth: Learn to speechread (lipread) and you will understand just fine.

Truth: Many people benefit from taking speechreading lessons; however speechreading is not a substitute for hearing aids but a complement to them. Research studies have found that only about three out of ten words can be speechread clearly, only about 30 to 40 percent of speech is visible, and many words that are visible look the same on the lips.

4

HOW YOUR HEARING LOSS AFFECTS YOUR FAMILY AND FRIENDS

Think about the many activities you enjoy with your family and friends and what it would be like to feel left out. Holiday gatherings, where everyone is talking at the same time, can become a frustrating and sad experience for you. While others are enjoying conversing with one another, you are missing out. You want to hear what your family members are talking about but cannot understand them and may have even more difficulty understanding what your grandchildren are saying.

You also may have curtailed other family activities including movies, watching television, playing cards, and eating out, which once were enjoyable family times, because you don't hear as well as you once did. Traveling, which includes understanding directions, information from tour guides, and conversation with strangers may become a source of anxiety rather than the fun it is supposed to be. Even conversing while driving a car, something you have enjoyed for years, becomes impossible.

When you lose your hearing, you lose your ability to communicate as easily as you once did. You do not lose your mind, your intelligence, your talent, or your sense of humor. This is important to remember, since the longer you deny you have a hearing loss, the more difficult it will be to maintain the relationships you have had with family and friends.

Family and friends are your sources of support. They will be there to work with you and stand by you when you

11

need them, but you need to do your part to earn their love and support.

Bluffing, in an effort to hide your hearing loss, often creates stressful situations for you and your family. When communication breaks down, tension, frustration, and anxiety often result. Misunderstandings occur, which can create problems such as missed appointments and confused directions and other information.

Hearing loss can drive you and your family apart. But it doesn't need to be that way.

What You Can Do

Sit down with family and friends and talk honestly. Admit that you have a hearing loss. Family members may initiate this talk because they have noticed the loss before you did. Tell them how you feel about your loss and what they can do to help. Perhaps you are self-conscious, or feel left out. You may be worried about losing even more hearing. You may be concerned about wearing a hearing aid, if a diagnosis suggests this recourse.

If you have not had your hearing loss diagnosed, this should be the first step (see Key 11). You and your family will want to know what kind of loss you have and what can be done about it. Most families have never dealt with a hearing loss and may have misconceptions about what to do. You and your family should learn about the many things you and they can do together to help you hear better and improve communication at home.

If the diagnosis suggests amplification—and this is not the answer for everyone—see a hearing health care specialist and together decide which is the best hearing aid for you (see Key 16). You will have taken the first step to improving communication.

You will need your family's support as you adjust to wearing the aid. Often, families think that a hearing aid will restore your hearing to normal. As you learn about the effects of background noise on your ability to hear with and without a hearing aid, you will need to let your family know what you are going through and what they can do to help.

You will need to educate your family about the best environments for communicating with you and changes such as lighting and positioning that should be made to enhance your understanding of speech. You also can give them tips for communicating with you (see Key 24).

If you are married, your spouse is the person most affected by your hearing loss. Your spouse may have known you when you could hear and may need to be reeducated as to the best way to communicate with you. Spouses will talk to you from another room, talk to your back, and even suggest that "you hear what you want to hear." You will need to be patient as you deal not only with your own hearing loss, but your spouse's frustrations as well. Pillow talk, an important part of your relationship, may no longer take place in the dark since you need to see your spouse's face in order to hear. The quality of your relationship will be enhanced as you make concerted efforts to work at communicating better.

It may be easy to let a family member with normal hearing do the talking and thus take over your life, but your quality of life is likely to suffer. Instead, avoid depending on your spouse or other family member by taking charge of the information you want to receive and share with others. Be careful not to confer the role of full-time interpreter on your spouse.

Family members often forget that you don't hear as well as you once did. It is okay to remind them about ways to communicate better. You will need to be patient and understanding but also assertive (see Key 23). Remember, taking control of your life and your rights without infringing on the rights of others is what honest and assertive communication is all about.

5

HOW THE EAR WORKS

The human ear is a delicate and sensitive structure. Under normal conditions it processes a wide range of acoustical activity through the nervous system and the brain in order for you to be able to hear sound.

When any part of the ear breaks down, it affects our ability to perceive sound. Disease, heredity, infections, and noise are among the causes of hearing loss. Aging (presbycusis) is another major cause of hearing deterioration.

To understand what happens when our hearing diminishes, you need to understand the anatomy of the ear and how it works.

Anatomy of the Ear

The ear has three major parts: the outer ear, the middle ear, and the inner ear (see Figure 2). The outer ear collects sound waves and funnels them into the middle ear, which passes them on to the inner ear. The inner ear converts the waves into nerve impulses and transmits them to the brain. The inner ear also contains the balance mechanism.

- The **outer ear** includes both the ear we see—the pinna—and the outer ear canal, a passage about three quarters of an inch long. Sound travels through the canal and hits the eardrum, a thin membrane that separates the outer ear from the middle ear.
- The **middle ear** is a small cavity between the eardrum and the inner ear. It contains three small, connected bones (ossicles): the malleus (hammer), the incus (anvil), and the stapes (stirrup). When the eardrum vibrates, these bones also vibrate, thus conducting sound to the inner ear. The middle ear also includes the

eustachian tube, which leads to the nose and throat, and whose main function is to keep the air pressure in the middle ear equal to the surrounding environment.

- The **inner ear** consists of two structures that contain membrane-lined chambers filled with fluid: the *labyrinth* and the *cochlea*. The labyrinth is the part of the ear used for balance. The cochlea plays a role in hearing. The auditory nerve attaches to the labyrinth and the cochlea, and connects the hearing and balance functions of the inner ear to appropriate parts of the brain. As sound vibrations are transmitted to the cochlea, they set tiny hair cells in motion. These hair cells transform the vibrations into nerve impulses. The acoustic nerve picks up these impulses and sends them to the brain, which interprets these signals as words and other sounds.

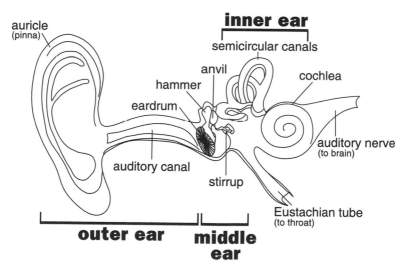

Figure 2 Anatomy of the Ear.

The labyrinth in each inner ear monitors the position and movements of the head by means of three semicircular canals. Each canal is at right angles to the other two so that when you nod, shake, or tilt your head, one or more of the canals detects the movement and relays the information to the brain. The brain, in turn, coordinates this information with your eyes and the muscles in your body to assess your exact position and the movements you need to make to keep your balance. When you experience a loss of balance, it usually means that you have a disorder of the inner ear.

Most sound starts outside the ear causing the air to vibrate and produce sound waves. The pinna channels the sound waves down the ear canal to the eardrum, which begins to vibrate. The vibrations pass through the hammer, anvil, stirrup, and oval window into the cochlea. The tiny hairs in the cochlea change the vibrations into nerve impulses, which are transmitted by the auditory nerve to the brain.

You will experience a hearing loss when sound cannot be transmitted normally through the ear canal because of an occlusion such as earwax, a perforated eardrum, damaged or defective ossicles, or damaged hair cells.

No matter what the nature of your hearing loss, a hearing health care specialist can conduct a painless evaluation and recommend the best treatment.

6

TYPES OF HEARING LOSS

Once you are aware that you have a hearing loss, you will want to learn more about it. Although sensorineural hearing loss is the most prevalent type of loss, especially in older people, you should seek a proper diagnosis from an appropriate hearing health care provider.

Sensorineural hearing loss. The most common cause of sensorineural hearing loss is aging, although high fevers, ototoxic drugs, and noise are other causes. If you have this type of hearing loss, you have trouble hearing in crowded rooms and while watching television, as well as difficulty understanding conversation. Also called *nerve deafness*, this type of hearing loss usually is not caused by damage to the auditory nerve but to the hair cells in the inner ear. The hair cells, which are tuned in for specific sounds, may be so severely damaged that they cannot react when sound from the outside strikes them. At the same time, hair cells for certain speech sounds may be functioning normally. This causes you to miss parts of words and sentences. Although rarely correctable medically or surgically, fortunately, in the great majority of cases, properly fitted hearing aids and assistive devices can help you hear better.

Conductive hearing loss. With conductive hearing loss, sounds seem soft but speech is clear as long as it is loud enough. This type of hearing loss is caused by a blockage that prevents sound from being conducted to the inner ear. The blockage can be caused by wax buildup, an ear infection, a fusion of the bones in the middle ear, or a punctured eardrum. This type of hearing loss often responds to medical or surgical treatment. You must, however, have

17

good function of the nerve and inner ear. When this is not possible, in some cases a hearing aid also can help.

Mixed hearing loss. This involves both conductive and sensorineural components. Medical or surgical intervention may help the conductive portion and a hearing aid can help the sensorineural loss.

Other Hearing Disorders

Other conditions often associated with hearing loss follow.

Tinnitus is the name for a ringing in the ears or other head noises, a common disorder experienced by nearly 36 million Americans. Tinnitus, which almost always accompanies a hearing loss, can also affect people with normal hearing. It may come and go, or it can be a constant companion. It can vary in pitch; it can affect one ear or both. Although for most people it presents no problem, tinnitus is annoying, and for some, so debilitating that it can prevent people who are affected from leading normal lives.

Ménière's disease is one of the more common causes of dizziness (vertigo). Its symptoms also include tinnitus and hearing loss fluctuation. Its cause is unknown but probably results from abnormality in the fluids of the inner ear. Currently, no known cure for Ménière's disease is available; however, medications can be prescribed for acute attacks, and symptoms may be somewhat reduced by adopting a low-sodium diet, avoiding caffeine and alcohol, stopping smoking, avoiding noisy and stressful situations, and using exercise to reduce stress and improve circulation. Sometimes surgery is recommended to relieve acute attacks of dizziness.

Other conditions. For information about other conditions associated with hearing loss such as otosclerosis, acoustic neuroma, Usher's Syndrome, and Cogan's Syndrome, consult your otolaryngologist and library resources.

7

CAUSES OF HEARING LOSS

There are many causes of hearing loss, including:
- heredity
- head injury
- diseases such as measles, mumps, and spinal meningitis
- noise
- aging (presbycusis)

If you recognized your hearing loss when you were 55 or older, the most probable cause was age-related hearing loss.

Heredity*. A large proportion of hearing loss that occurs at birth or in the first few years of life is hereditary. Many types of adult-onset and progressive hearing loss are also hereditary. A hereditary (genetic) hearing loss is sometimes easy to identify from family history; a parent or a sibling also may have a loss. In some families, however, the gene that causes hearing loss is recessive, which means the hearing loss may be passed on by parents, even if they themselves do not have a hearing loss.

Accidents. Accidents causing head injury can cause a dramatic hearing loss. It is usually sudden and traumatic.

Maternal rubella. Although not as prevalent as it once was since the inception of vaccinations to prevent maternal rubella (the mother had German measles during pregnancy), this was a major cause of hearing loss in people born in the mid-1960s.

---

*The National Institute on Deafness and Other Communication Disorders (NIDCD) has established a Hereditary Hearing Impairment Resource Registry. The registry, a directory of families who have at least one member with a hearing loss, was established to help scientists doing research in hereditary hearing loss. For more information, see Appendix B.

Disease. Diseases such as measles, mumps, and spinal meningitis that are accompanied by high fever have been the cause of hearing loss in many people.

Aging. Presbycusis is the term used to describe the slow, progressive type of hearing loss that is associated with aging. At age 65, one out of every three people has a hearing loss. Age-related hearing loss often is due to a lifetime of exposure to dangerous levels of noise (see below) or to hereditary adult-onset hearing loss.

Noise. Prolonged exposure to loud noise at or above 90 decibels can damage the sensitive hair cells lining the cochlea. This may cause partial or severe hearing loss. Occupational noise exposure, the most common form of noise-induced hearing loss, threatens the hearing of firefighters, police officers, military personnel, construction and factory workers, musicians, farmers, and truck drivers, to name a few. Nonoccupational sources of hazardous noise such as live or recorded high volume music; recreational vehicles; airplanes; lawn-care equipment; woodworking tools; household appliances such as mixers, blenders, and vacuum cleaners; and chain saws also cause hearing loss. Because no medical or surgical treatment can correct a hearing loss resulting from noise exposure, prevention is important.

Drugs. Some drugs prescribed for medical problems are ototoxic, meaning they have the potential to cause damage to the inner ear, which may result in temporary or permanent hearing loss. If you have a hearing loss, ask your doctor about the medications prescribed for you so that you can prevent an aggravation of your hearing problem (see Key 8).

Unfortunately, many cases of hearing loss are due to unknown causes.

8

EFFECT OF MEDICATION ON HEARING LOSS

Ototoxic medications are drugs that may cause damage to the inner ear resulting in temporary or permanent hearing loss and tinnitus. If you have a sensorineural hearing loss, you should ask your doctor and pharmacist about medications prescribed for you since you will want to prevent an aggravation of your hearing problem.

The degree of hearing loss that you experience when taking an ototoxic drug depends on the amount and duration of the use of the medication. If you are taking more than one ototoxic medication, you are even more vulnerable to developing a sensorineural hearing loss or aggravating your existing hearing loss. With many drugs, such as aspirin, hearing loss returns to normal after they are discontinued, no matter how much or how long you use them.

If you experience any of the following signs of ototoxicity, consult your doctor. Some common symptoms are:
- noises in your ear (tinnitus)
- pressure in your ears
- an awareness of, and a fluctuation or increase in the degree of your hearing loss
- dizziness

Tell your doctor about your hearing loss and ask if any of the medications prescribed are ototoxic. Ask your pharmacist if any over-the-counter medications you buy have ototoxic effects. Your hearing health care specialist also needs to know about drugs you are taking that may cause fluctuations in your hearing or changes in auditory perception.

Common Ototoxic Medications

Some common ototoxic medications and their effects follow.

Salicylates. The ototoxic effects of aspirin and aspirin-containing products appear after taking six to eight pills per day. Toxic effects are always reversible once medication is discontinued.

Nonsteroidal anti-inflammatory drugs. The ototoxic effects of NSAIDS such as Advil and Aleve, Clinoril, and Motrin appear after taking six to eight pills per day. Toxic effects are usually reversible once the medication is discontinued.

Antibiotics. Drugs such as streptomycin, erythromycin, and vancomycin when given intravenously are ototoxic. When used topically or administered orally, these drugs are not known to cause hearing loss.

Loop diuretics. Medications such as Lasix, Edecrin, and Bumex are usually ototoxic when administered intravenously. Ototoxicity is rare when these drugs are given orally.

Chemotherapeutic agents. Medications such as cisplatin, nitrogen mustard, and vincristine are ototoxic when given for treatment of cancer. The ototoxic effects are enhanced if you are already taking other ototoxic medications such as aminoglycoside antibiotics (streptomycin, kanamycin, neomycin, gentamycin, tobramycin, amikacin, netilmycin) and loop diuretics.

Quinine. The ototoxic effects of drugs containing quinine, such as aralen, atabrine, legatrin, and Q-Vel muscle relaxant, are similar to those of aspirin. The toxic effects are usually reversible once medication is discontinued.

Being aware of ototoxic medications and their early warning signs is important in preserving your residual hearing. If you experience any of the signs of ototoxicity mentioned above, stop the medication immediately and call your doctor.

9

NOISE

One of the more frequent complaints made by hard of hearing people is difficulty hearing in noisy surroundings. What may be an acceptable noise level for a person with normal hearing can completely obliterate speech comprehension for someone who is hard of hearing. From this point of view, noise is as much an environmental pollutant as secondary smoke.

Few places exist today that can shield you from loud environmental sounds. Machinery, traffic noise, impact noise, and blast sounds from weapons and detonation exact a heavy toll on fragile, specialized cells, known as hair cells, within the inner ear. Exposure to excessive noise is a leading cause of hearing loss, and such hearing loss is irreversible.

The first signs of noise-induced hearing loss are typically decreased hearing at higher frequencies (3000–6000 Hz), that part of the frequency range in which many of the important consonant sounds lie. You may notice that you cannot distinguish between *back* and *bat* and *flip* and *trip*. With time, noise-induced hearing loss also erodes mid-frequency, and later, low-frequency hearing.

The potential for noise to damage the ear depends on the intensity, tonal qualities, and duration of exposure. The louder, more continuous, and monotonous the noise, the more damage it does. Lawn mowers, leaf blowers, and power saws can cause hearing loss. Common household equipment such as vacuum cleaners and stereos can damage your hearing. Noise in factories, on the farm, and on the street are all harmful to your hearing. Even recreational activities such as hunting, motorcycling, and snowmobiling can cause a loss of hearing.

The effects of moderately loud sounds, such as small engines, can accumulate over years and lead to progressive degeneration of the inner ear's hair cells. Extremely loud sounds, such as the noise from rock concerts, large construction equipment, and blasts, may do damage by tearing delicate inner ear membranes.

If you already have some degree of hearing loss, it is especially important to protect your residual hearing. While it is true that your hearing loss protects you against some loud noises, if the noise is intense enough that it sounds loud to you despite your hearing loss, your ears are probably more sensitive, and you could develop a noise-induced hearing loss. If you know that you are going to be exposed to loud sounds, take no chances—wear hearing protection to avoid further loss.

What else can you do to protect yourself? You can control the noise in your home by turning down the volume on the radio, TV, and stereo, and by using audio headsets only when necessary. You can protect yourself from noise by wearing earplugs, earmuffs, or both. Earplugs can be specially made to custom fit your ear canals, and newer designs let in some speech and music sounds. An audiologist can provide information on the options for hearing protection.

An unwelcome fact is that each day many of us lose a little of our ability to hear because of noise surrounding us. In our homes, in the workplace, and on the street, we regularly expose ourselves to dangerous noise levels. In our recreation, too, when we turn to music, one of society's main sources of entertainment, we endanger our hearing by listening to music at dangerously high levels. And as we age, our hearing loss may very well be attributed to a lifetime of exposure to dangerous levels of noise.

10

WHAT TO DO IF YOU SUSPECT A HEARING LOSS

Hearing loss is not in itself a disease. It is a symptom of some underlying disorder. Some hearing loss is common as you get older, but if you are under 50 and notice you have a hearing loss, you should see an otolaryngologist or an audiologist, who is trained to identify symptoms that should be treated by a physician. The treatment may be something as simple as flushing out your ears to remove a wax buildup.

If a doctor determines that your hearing loss is not correctable by medication or surgery, you should see a trained specialist for a hearing evaluation. The hearing evaluation will determine if you have a hearing loss, the extent of the loss, and what you can do to hear better.

The person who performs the evaluation is as important as the evaluation itself. You should choose this person carefully (see Key 12).

There are three kinds of hearing health care providers: otolaryngologists, audiologists, and hearing aid specialists.

Otolaryngologists (ear, nose, and throat specialists) are physicians who provide medical and surgical treatment for hearing disorders. If your condition cannot be treated medically or surgically, a hearing evaluation is the next step. These physicians do not normally dispense hearing aids; many of them, however, employ audiologists to evaluate your hearing loss and dispense them.

Audiologists have a minimum of a master's degree in the evaluation and nonmedical treatment of hearing loss. They are licensed in 38 states, and many are certified by the American Association of Speech-Language-Pathology and Audiology (ASHA). Most audiologists also fit and dispense hearing aids. The audiologist can determine the type and degree of hearing loss and whether or not you can be helped by a hearing aid (or aids), and if so, what type of hearing aid would be best for you.

Hearing aid specialists (also called hearing aid dealers) are licensed in all but four states to test hearing and sell hearing aids. While these dealers have less formal education and do not provide diagnostic audiological services, some have considerable experience. In many areas, hearing aid specialists are the only hearing health care specialists available.

Make sure that whomever you choose is someone who spends adequate time informing and counseling you and in whom you have confidence and trust.

In addition to consulting professionals, begin to educate yourself about hearing loss. Go to the library and read everything you can find about hearing loss. Talk to friends who have a hearing loss or know someone who does. Learn strategies for coping with hearing loss and use them. These may make a difference in your ability to understand what is being said even before you see a hearing health care specialist.

In 250 SHHH local chapters across the country, people meet monthly to learn from one another about successful strategies for living with hearing loss. Meeting other people who have a hearing loss helps you realize that you are not alone. Peer support helps you learn about hearing loss and ways to live with it.

11

UNDERSTANDING YOUR HEARING EVALUATION

Whether you have had your hearing tested many times before or are preparing for your first evaluation, a hearing assessment can be confusing and even overwhelming. You receive so much new information that you may find it hard to process everything.

Understanding what happens during a hearing evaluation and how that information relates to your communication abilities makes it possible for you to be an informed and active participant in shaping your hearing health care. In addition, you will be better equipped to judge whether you are receiving good, appropriate, and ethical service.

A hearing health care provider (audiologist or hearing aid specialist) begins the evaluation by taking a case history. You will be asked about your hearing loss, situations in which you find it difficult to hear, and what you are not hearing. You will take a battery of tests to determine the extent of your hearing loss and your understanding of speech. Don't forget to tell the tester about any medication you take regularly, especially ones that might be ototoxic.

All audiometric tests should be performed in a sound-proof booth. Only in rare cases, such as when patients are bedridden, should they be performed in homes or elsewhere.

The tester either places earphones over your ears or uses a loudspeaker to send sounds to one or both ears. It is important that both ears be tested individually since the degree of hearing loss for each may differ. The tester will instruct you to raise your hand or a finger or push a button when you hear a sound.

The Hearing Evaluation

A complete hearing evaluation includes most of the following tests:

Pure tone air conduction. The tester measures your ability to hear different tones of sound, measured in hertz (Hz) and your ability to hear the loudness or intensity of these tones, measured in decibels (dB).

Speech reception and speech discrimination. Following the pure tone test, the evaluator adjusts the volume and frequency to test your understanding (discrimination). This is done by using various kinds of test stimuli, such as nonsense syllables, monosyllabic words, or sentences. If your discrimination is 70 percent, you cannot understand 30 percent of the words you hear. The greater your discrimination loss, the more difficulty you will have understanding in situations with background noise.

Pure-tone bone conduction. If the testing reveals that you have a hearing loss, the kind of loss is determined by using a bone vibrator. The bone vibrator sends sounds to the inner ear, bypassing the outer and middle ear. This test determines whether you have a conductive, sensorineural, or mixed hearing loss.

Threshold of discomfort, comfort, and awareness. Using connected speech stimuli, the tester measures your thresholds of speech awareness, comfort, and discomfort. These measures indicate your range of hearing (soft to loud) and provide important information when fitting a hearing aid.

Impedance testing. Impedance testing measures the ability of your eardrum to reflect sound waves. Too much or too little pressure on the inner side of the eardrum makes the eardrum too stiff to conduct and reflect sounds properly. The tester puts a probe covered with a soundproof material into your outer ear canal and seals up the entrance of the ear. A transmitter in the probe aims sounds at the eardrum. A receiver in the probe measures the reflections while air pumped through the probe changes the pressure in the canal rapidly from high to low. The test is one more way to determine whether the middle ear space is functioning normally.

The tester records your test results on an audiogram and then should explain the audiogram and its implications. At the beginning of your hearing evaluation, ask for a copy of your audiogram when it is completed. It is one of the first steps in understanding your hearing loss.

The Audiogram
The audiogram will give you a basic picture of your ability to detect tones. The tester plots your hearing threshold—the very softest sound you can detect at a particular frequency—on a grid, with frequency (Hz) on the horizontal axis and hearing level (dB) on the vertical axis. Circles are used to record the threshold for your right ear and Xs indicate the left ear thresholds. The louder that sound must be made to be barely heard represents the degree of hearing loss (see Figure 3).

Generally, Hz measurements start at 125 and increase in octave intervals up to 8000 Hz. Loudness is measured in 10 dB increments, starting at 0 dB at the top of the audiogram and progressing to 110+ dB.

The tester will determine whether you need amplification based on the results of your speech discrimination hearing test and your audiogram. If hearing aid(s) are recommended, be sure you learn about the various kinds of aids, how they will help you, what their limitations are, and how to buy them.

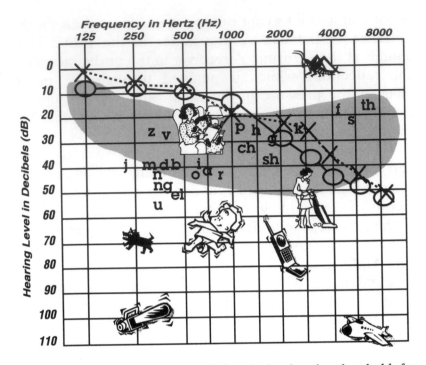

Figure 3 The audiogram is a graph that depicts hearing thresholds for selected tones (Hz) at various intensities (dB). The circles mark the lowest intensity at which the right ear picks up tones, while the Xs show the thresholds for the left ear. The shaded area indicates the tones and intensities that individuals generally need to hear in order to recognize parts of speech clearly. The letters show the Hz and dB levels where individual speech sounds are heard, and the pictographs show the range of some common sounds. On an audiogram provided by your hearing health provider, the Xs and circles are usually depicted in different colors for clarity. Chris Blum/*Hearing Health Magazine,* Ingleside, Texas. Reprinted with permission.

12

CHOOSING A HEARING HEALTH CARE DISPENSER

If your hearing evaluation determines that amplification will help you hear better, you will have the important job of selecting a hearing health care dispenser. This step is extremely important since you are choosing a person with whom you will have a long-term relationship, and, as in all relationships, you will want this to be comfortable and mutually beneficial.

The best way to find a responsive dispenser is to talk to friends and relatives who wear hearing aids, are comfortable with them, and have had a positive experience during the selection, purchase, and aural rehabilitation program.

Selecting the right hearing aid takes time and patience. Not only will you have several visits with a hearing health care dispenser before the final purchase, you will return again and again for evaluations, repairs, education, and, eventually, new hearing aids.

You should expect the following skills, attitudes, and services from the hearing aid dispenser:

1. **Interpersonal skills.** Look for a person who is courteous and patient and willing to listen to you. The dispenser should see you as a person with a hearing loss, but one that has an individual lifestyle.
2. **Competency.** Be sure that the dispenser is licensed or certified, keeps up with the latest advances in hearing aids and fitting, and makes excellent earmold impressions.
3. **Adequate diagnostic and testing equipment.** The dispenser should perform tests in a soundproof room, have up-to-date testing equipment, and should provide

you with an explanation of the results as well as a copy of your audiogram.

4. **Selection assistance.** The dispenser should explain clearly the difference in hearing aids and their performance and have a variety of brands and styles for you to try out in different communication situations such as on the telephone, and in a noisy location. The dispenser also should provide information about options beyond the hearing aid, including assistive devices.

5. **Education and rehabilitation services.** The dispenser should describe how the aid functions as well as its limitations. When you receive your hearing aid, the dispenser should conduct a training session and follow up at periodic intervals to ensure your satisfaction. Some dispensers provide group hearing aid evaluation orientation sessions and evaluation for hearing assistive technology. If your dispenser does not offer an aural rehabilitation program, ask for help in finding one.

6. **Pricing and service policies.** The dispenser should clearly explain all the costs that you can expect and which fees are nonrefundable if you need to return the aid. Typically, costs for testing, custom-fit parts, and earmolds, are nonrefundable. You should expect to have at least a 30-day (preferably 60-day) trial period to try out the aid (this is the law in some states). This gives you time to "test-drive" the aid, just as you would when buying a new car. The dispenser should provide repair service and give you a loaner free of charge should you need repair (see Key 16).

7. **Parking facilities and proximity to public transportation.** A dispenser whose facility is located near public transportation or has convenient parking may be a consideration for some older Americans.

Hearing aids are expensive. Don't be rushed into a decision. Choose a dispenser whose primary goal is to satisfy your needs.

13

WILL A
HEARING AID HELP?

A hearing aid will not correct or restore your hearing, but it will help you to hear by amplifying sounds. Most hearing aids have a manual volume control that allows you to increase or decrease the volume as needed. Some newer models have a built-in volume control (automatic signal processing) that does this automatically.

A hearing aid also will amplify most other sounds in your environment. Sometimes this is desirable since you want to hear the telephone and doorbell as well as other sounds that alert you to changes; however, hearing aids also will amplify dinnerware clanging and background noise in large group settings.

If you have trouble hearing and differentiating between certain sounds such as *f* and *s* (high-frequency sounds), your hearing aid can be set to increase the volume of those sounds, which can influence the clarity and help you hear better.

If you have difficulty hearing on the telephone, a hearing aid with a T-switch (telecoil) will enable you to use a variety of assistive technologies to improve your telephone communications (see Keys 17 and 19).

There are many manufacturers and many models of hearing aids and there are new models coming on the market every year. There is no "best" hearing aid. Each person has an individualized hearing loss; what is right for others may not be right for you. Just because someone you know is happy with his or her aid does not mean that it will work well for you. Hearing aid selection depends on many factors, including the degree of your hearing loss, your demands on hearing, your manual dexterity, the situations in which you communicate, and how much you can afford to spend.

Hearing aids are not comparable to eyeglasses, which can correct vision to normal. In fact, the sounds coming through the hearing aid can at first sound unnatural— tinny and mechanical. With continued use, the auditory system adapts to this new sound and it is then perceived to be more like "normal" sound. Many people who expect "normal" hearing through a new hearing aid are disappointed and, after a few brief trials, stick the aid in a bureau drawer permanently.

Also, when a hearing aid is first worn, some everyday sounds, such as footsteps, birds chirping, and paper shuffling, often are heard for the first time in years. These sounds may be disturbing or distracting, but with time and use of the hearing aid, the sounds become less disturbing and even enjoyable. However, when hearing aids are optimally fit, the brain can reorganize new sound patterns, which permits you to have increased sound perception. New hearing aid users need at least a six- to eight-week adjustment period to determine the full benefit.

Properly selected, properly fitted, and properly used with follow-up care, a hearing aid is a positive start to dealing with your hearing loss. The initial steps of coming to terms with not hearing well and getting a hearing aid need not be overwhelming. Many successful hearing aid users will tell you that a hearing aid has brought them out of isolation and greatly increased their independence and quality of life.

14

TYPES OF HEARING AIDS

All hearing aids work in a similar fashion and have similar parts. These include:

- a microphone to pick up sound
- an amplifier to make sound louder
- a receiver (miniature loudspeaker) to deliver the louder sound to the ear
- batteries to power the electronic parts

Some hearing aids also have earmolds to control the flow of sound into the ear, enhance sound quality, and help hold the hearing aid in place. Other hearing aids are built right into the earmold.

Hearing aids also differ in design, power, ease of handling, and availability of special features. You, in consultation with your hearing aid dispenser, should decide which of the many styles best meets your needs.

There are three major and three minor types of hearing aids in use today:

1. **In-the-canal (ITC) hearing aids** are contained in a tiny case that fits into the ear canal. If your hearing loss is mild and you hear well on the telephone, you may want to consider this model. However, if you have trouble with manual dexterity, consider a different model.

2. **In-the-ear (ITE) hearing aids** fit into the contour of the outer ear with a portion extending into the ear canal. They are larger and more visible than canal aids and can be used by people with hearing losses ranging from mild to moderate-severe. These models can include a telecoil. Some of the smaller ITE hearing aids are known as completely-in-the-canal (CIC) aids.

3. **Behind-the-ear (BTE) hearing aids** fit securely behind the ear and require an earmold worn in the outer ear that is connected by a tube and hook to the aid. BTEs are recommended for the entire range of hearing losses.
4. **Eyeglass-type hearing aids** have all parts of the aid fitted into the frames of your eyeglasses. Clear plastic tubing connects the bow to an earmold. Very few people currently wear this type of hearing aid.
5. **CROS (Contralateral Routing of Signal) and BICROS (Bilateral Routing of Signals)** are instruments designed to transmit sound from a microphone located near a nonfunctional ear to a receiver on the other ear. A CROS aid is used if the better ear has close to normal hearing; a BICROS aid is used if the better ear requires amplification in its own right.
6. **Body hearing aids** are large and very powerful aids that are used for profound hearing losses. All parts are contained in a case that is worn on the body (clipped to a bra or pocket); a cord connecting the case to the receiver runs along the neck and the receiver then snaps into an earmold with wires extending from the receiver to an earmold.

The newest generation of hearing aids are extremely sophisticated electronic devices. Some that are on the market are essentially minicomputers. They can be programmed and then reprogrammed to provide different kinds of amplification characteristics depending on your hearing loss, with some including a multiple-memory mode that can be modified as the listening situation changes. These hearing aids tend to be much more expensive than more conventional hearing aids and the cost-benefit ratio may not be sufficient to justify the extra expense. For this reason, it is important to have confidence in the skills and advice of your hearing aid dispenser, but still have the option to return the hearing aids after a trial period.

Binaural Hearing Aids

If you have a loss in both ears, your audiologist may recommend that you consider a binaural fitting (two hearing aids). There are many advantages to wearing two aids including hearing in noisy environments and determining from which direction a sound is coming. As is always the case with a hearing aid purchase, be sure you can return one aid at the end of the trial period, usually one month, if you are uncomfortable with two aids.

Hearing Aid Special Features

Two options to consider when selecting a hearing aid follow.

T-switch or telecoil. Some hearing aids have a switch that allows you to select microphone (M) or telecoil (T). Some aids also have a combination M-T-switch, which activates the telecoil and microphone simultaneously. Hearing aids incorporating a T-switch are often no more expensive if you request the switch at the time of testing or purchase. The T-switch is an option that can be included in all but the tiniest aids.

Direct audio input. Many models of behind-the-ear hearing aids are designed to accept direct audio input. An adapter shoe or boot connects the hearing aid receiver to an assistive listening device or to an external microphone via wire cords. This connection bypasses the hearing aid's microphone and can dramatically improve the signal-noise ratio. Some behind-the-ear and most in-the-ear canal aids do not permit direct audio input.

15

THE IMPORTANCE OF FITTING HEARING AIDS

When the testing and evaluation of your hearing determines that you can benefit from a hearing aid, the hearing aid dispenser will proceed with the proper fitting.

Making an Impression
The hearing aid dispenser will insert a soft waxlike material into your ear to make an impression of your ear canal and outer ear. This is an essential part of the hearing aid fitting. If you decide to purchase an in-the-ear (ITE) or in-the-canal (ITC) aid, this step is extremely important because, if not done properly, the aid will not fit correctly. If you decide to purchase a behind-the-ear (BTE) aid, you also will need an impression in order to have an earmold made.

Earmolds
The purpose of the earmold is to couple the sound from your hearing aid to your ear. The degree and configuration of your hearing loss determines the type of earmold you need. There are many different kinds of earmolds and it is important to have the kind that is right for you. The hearing aid dispenser will send the impression to a laboratory where it is copied in a hard (acrylic) or soft (polyvinyl) synthetic material. Nonallergenic polyethylene is recommended for people who have allergic reactions to the other two.

When the earmold is returned from the manufacturer, the dispenser will ensure that the fit is tight so that all amplified sound goes into your ear. An earmold that is too small causes feedback (whistling or squealing), or you may hear an echo when you speak, or the sound may be distorted. One that is too large will not fit or may be uncomfortable. Sometimes the dispenser can file it to fit; however, if that does not work, you should expect the impression and earmold to be remade at no additional cost.

If you consider trying a BTE, the hearing aid dispenser will connect the mold to several different BTE hearing aids and you will begin the selection of one that is best for you. The dispenser may try several models of one brand or several different brands before you both can decide which one helps you most in the environments where you will need it most.

If you decide to try an ITE or ITC, the impression taken for the mold is used to construct the hearing aid. This is why a good earmold impression is always essential.

Once you have selected a hearing aid, the dispenser will evaluate your hearing with the aid in place and measure the increased benefit you receive from the aid, keeping appropriate records so that you are always able to compare your current situation to a previous one.

Feedback

Feedback occurs when some of the amplified sound escapes from around the earmold or the ITE or ITC aid, gets picked up by the hearing aid microphone, and then reamplified to start the process all over again. Some feedback is normal, such as when you cup your hand over your ear, if you remove your aid without turning it off, or if you lie down with your aid turned on. However, if you get feedback when you chew or smile, or when you turn the volume higher, it may be a sign that the mold or aid does not fit well.

Replacing the Mold

Since the ear is made of cartilage, it is always changing in shape and size. At the same time, vinyl materials tend to shrink over time. You, therefore, should have your mold checked regularly to determine if you need a new one. If the mold has become discolored or hard, it's time to get a new one.

Cleaning the Earmold

Each evening, when you remove your hearing aid, you should wipe the earmold with a tissue. If you have a problem with earwax clogging the mold, this step is even more important because the smallest amount of wax can affect the sound reception. If the earmold can be removed from the aid, you can soak it in warm dishwashing liquid and water once a week. Dry it carefully before attaching it to the aid. A small rubber ball syringe will remove the moisture from the tubing. Do not use alcohol or other chemicals to clean your earmold since they may cause it to crack. Nonallergenic material may need to be washed more often, as it tends to grip in the ear canal, sponging up earwax and dirt.

Wax

Earwax or *cerumen* is the body's natural way of lubricating the ear canal and keeping insects out of it since they do not like the odor; however, wax may obstruct the canal so that sound does not pass through clearly. For that reason it is important to have a doctor remove the wax from your ear canals before you are evaluated for a hearing loss. Wax also can clog earmold openings or plug up vents in hearing aids, so these should be checked daily. You can clean small amounts of wax from the earmold or tubing with a pipe cleaner or the tool provided by the hearing aid manufacturer.

16

PURCHASING A HEARING AID

Be an Educated Consumer

Selecting the right hearing aid for purchase is an important decision. It also can be stressful, especially if it is your first hearing aid. With other important purchases, such as automobiles and refrigerators, we can depend on recommendations from friends who have had good experiences with those products. But since each person's hearing loss is individualized, the make and model of a hearing aid that works well for your friend may not be beneficial to you.

Becoming an educated consumer is key to your success in choosing the right hearing aid. Your hearing aid dispenser should point out the pros and cons of various aids in terms of ease of handling, comfort, and suitability based on your hearing loss. You, in turn, must state your specific needs and wants. The final choice should emerge from your responses while trying several makes and models and considering the advantages and disadvantages of each.

Although hearing aids last for four or more years, they are expensive. The average price for hearing aids follows:

Programmable aid	$1563
In-the-canal aid	$952
In-the-ear aid	$762
Behind-the-ear aid	$765

The newest generation of programmable digital hearing aids may cost as much as $2500. These prices, in most instances, include testing and fitting.

Many hearing aid dispensers include testing in the price of the hearing aid, while others do not. When testing fees

41

are separate, the hearing aid should cost less. Find out what services the costs include.

Ask about various options available in the hearing instrument such as a T-switch or direct audio input (see Key 14). These cost less when included at the time of purchase.

When you purchase a hearing aid, be sure to get a purchase agreement or sales contract containing all the terms of the transaction in writing, and read it carefully. It should include the following items:

Price. Prices vary depending on the kind and model, where you purchase the aid, and what services are provided. This is one good reason to ask what the price includes.

Payment agreement. Your contract should explain the payment terms in detail, including such items as down payment, interest, other charges, and insurance coverage.

Trial period. The normal trial period for a hearing aid is 30 days. During this period, you may return the aid for any reason, provided it is in good condition. The trial period should be explained up front. Be sure you know whether 30 days means calendar or working days. If you are offered or can negotiate a longer trial period, by all means do so since it takes some time for the brain to adjust to the new sounds you will be hearing.

What is refundable? You may have to pay a rental fee for the 30-day trial period; if you decide to purchase the aid, the rental fee should be refunded. If you purchase a BTE aid, you will be charged a fee for making the earmold. This fee is nonrefundable; however, the earmolds are yours to keep.

Rehabilitation services. Most new users need training and help adjusting to hearing aids. You may need two or three visits after you get your new aid to ensure that you are getting maximum benefit and understand its potential. With the newer programmable aids, you may need even more visits. If your hearing health care specialist offers group rehabilitation sessions, be sure to enroll. Learning to be a successful hearing aid user requires practice. This service is an important part of your contract.

Warranty. Almost all hearing aids carry a one- or two-year warranty for defects in material or workmanship. Most warranties do not cover external receivers, cords, earmolds, tubing, or batteries. Some offer a one-year loss and damage policy. Read over the warranty and inquire whether it is honored by the dispenser, the manufacturer, or both. You may wish to mark your calendar on a date several weeks before the warranty expires to remind you to be sure that the aid is in good working order.

Insurance coverage. Your health care plan, medicare, or medicaid may cover costs for a hearing test and hearing aid evaluation, but very few insurance policies cover the cost of hearing aids. Medicare doesn't cover them at all. Medicaid, which is restricted to eligible participants, provides for one aid only, with upper limits on the cost. Inquire whether insurance coverage against damage or loss is an option and if it is included in the cost of the aid.

Other Costs to Consider

Consider the following costs when purchasing an aid.

Batteries. Different aids use different sizes and types of batteries. Find out which batteries are used in your model, how long they last, and how much they cost. The length of time batteries last depends on how much you use the aid and at what power.

Repairs. Hearing aids sometimes need to be repaired. If your hearing aid malfunctions, it is best to take it to the dispenser for proper diagnosis and advice. The dispenser may be able to fix the aid at less cost to you and may offer you a loaner; major repairs may take longer. The cost of the repair service (out of warranty) usually includes a three- or six-month warranty. When the warranty and service plan expire, you will need to pay for repairs.

Other Options for Payment

Many civic and service organizations recondition hearing aids and put them in the hands of people who need them. Speech and hearing centers may provide hearing aids at a reduced rate for clients who patronize them. Hear Now provides aids to people who need them and also welcomes donations of used hearing aids (see Appendix B). All World War I veterans are eligible to receive free hearing aids. The eligibility of other veterans is decided on a case-by-case basis. Vocational Rehabilitation provides services for clients who meet eligibility requirements.

Note: Never purchase a hearing aid by mail or by phone. Remember that you are not only purchasing a device but also the services of a specialist, who will test the fit and fine tune the aid when needed, and advise you.

17

WHEN HEARING AIDS ARE NOT ENOUGH

While hearing aids are beneficial to many people, they may need to be supplemented in some situations. Even with hearing aids, people with hearing loss may have a great deal of difficulty understanding speech in noisy situations or when the sound source is some distance from them.

If you are unable to hear well at ceremonies relating to celebrations of life—such as weddings, baptisms, bar mitzvahs, and funerals—your hearing loss may be creating a barrier that could result in a deep sense of deprivation and loss. If you are reluctant to participate in community and congregational life because you cannot hear well, you may be needlessly isolating yourself from activities. Nevertheless, if the meeting and lecture rooms you frequent are not equipped with special sound systems, thus making dialogue inaccessible to you, don't give up.

In recent years, the technology designed to supplement hearing aids has burgeoned. New devices are developed, improved, and marketed each year. Two general types have been developed: assistive listening devices (ALDs), which include, but are not limited to, telephone listening devices (see Key 19); and various kinds of signaling and warning devices (see Key 18).

Assistive Listening Devices
All assistive listening devices enhance hearing in everyday situations by reducing the negative effects of distance, background noise, and reverberations. They do

this by transmitting the sound from the source via a microphone, movie sound track, or other external sound source directly to the ears of a listener. An electromagnetic field, radio wave, or infrared light beam transmits the sound directly to the ears of the person with a hearing loss via a special receiver. Choosing the right assistive listening device requires careful thought. The best way to choose an ALD is to assess your needs, discuss them with your hearing health care professional, and try out the devices available.

Personal Amplifiers
Sometimes called one-on-one communicators, these acoustic amplifiers include a built-in microphone and an amplifier and can accommodate most types of headphones. They are particularly helpful in small group situations when background noise interferes with your ability to understand the speaker. You may find these helpful in restaurants, at small group meetings, and in the car when you and the driver wish to keep your eyes on the road.

Large-Area Assistive Listening Systems
You also should learn about large-area assistive listening systems for improved listening in large rooms of assembly, places of worship, museums, theaters and movies, convention centers, public agency meeting rooms, and corporate conference rooms. Wireless assistive listening systems are divided into three primary types: Audio induction loop, infrared, and FM.

Audio induction loop system. The audio induction loop is a coil of electrical wire that is placed around a selected area. The wire, which creates a magnetic field that can transmit sound, is connected to an amplifier and to the speaker's microphone, TV, tape recorder, or other sound source. It differs from a public address system in that the amplified signal is sent to the coil of wire rather than to the loudspeakers. The magnetic field around the wire is picked up by individuals who wear hearing aids equipped with a telecoil (T-switch). The signal also can be picked up with a headset and receiver if the hard of hearing person is not wearing a hearing aid. The hard of hearing person can sit anywhere inside or alongside the loop and hear the sound without the disturbing effects of background noise or echoes.

Infrared system. This system is often found in theaters, courtrooms, and other public facilities. It uses an invisible light beam to transmit sound. The hard of hearing person wears a headset with a receiver that is in a direct line with the infrared light beam. Listeners who wear hearing aids with a T-switch can wear a neck loop plugged into the receiver or a silhouette behind the ear. An infrared system can only be used indoors.

FM (Frequency Modulation) system. The Federal Communications Commission has designated certain radio frequencies for use by people with hearing loss. The speaker wears a microphone connected to a small FM transmitter worn on the belt or around the neck, while the hard of hearing person wears an FM receiver connected to earphones or personal hearing aids. The transmitter and the receiver need to be set to the same radio frequency. Personal FM systems can be used to help in any situation where it is possible to place the microphone close to the sound source, such as in a noisy restaurant, moving car, small meetings, and near a TV loudspeaker. FM systems also can be used for listening in large areas, such as classrooms, auditoriums, movie houses, and places of worship. These are the kinds of places where hard of hearing people typically have a great deal of difficulty understanding speech. A "large-area" FM transmitter can be hooked into an existing P.A. system, using the same type of FM receiver that personal FM systems do. They work extremely well in delivering a clear speech signal to hard of hearing people in these stressful listening conditions.

Television Listening Devices
Television has become our window on the world; when we cannot hear and understand TV, we are frustrated. When we turn the volume up in order to hear what is amplified through the loudspeakers, the noise can be disturbing to others. Several TV listening devices (loops, FM, infrared) are available to enable a person who is hard of hearing to hear without turning the volume too loud for other listeners. The principle is the same as with large-area listening systems: The sound is picked up from the TV set (by placing a microphone close to the loudspeaker, or plugging the listening device into an audio output jack). The TV sound is then transmitted directly to the ears of the person wearing the hearing device.

Closed Captions
In addition to TV listening devices, you may want to consider captions if you are having difficulty understanding what is being said on television. Closed captions are the text display of spoken dialogue and sounds that are visible with the use of a decoder. All new TV sets larger than 13 inches come with built-in closed caption chips that can be activated to show captions when desired. Older TV sets can be connected to separate telecaption decoders, which operate to present the same closed-caption message. Nearly all prime-time television programming for major networks is closed captioned for hard of hearing and deaf people.

18

HEARING THE DOORBELL, TELEPHONE, AND FIRE ALARM

Signaling Devices

You may find that you have difficulty hearing a ringing doorbell or telephone, a knock on the door, a smoke or fire alarm, an alarm clock, a baby's cry, and other sounds that alert people to daily life occurrences. Fortunately, signaling devices are available to help compensate for your hearing loss and allow you to gain a greater sense of confidence and security at home, on the job, and while traveling.

The principle of all signaling devices is to detect sound by producing visual signals or vibrations that supplement auditory signals. Using the signaling equipment is a substitute for hearing the sound. The most common signaling device is a flashing light, but you may prefer a vibrating device placed under your pillow or mattress or under the cushion of your chair. Inexpensive systems are limited to one designated sound, but sophisticated systems are available that incorporate light patterns for various sounds.

Wake-up systems. Wake-up alarms include digital and standard clocks, bed vibrators, and timers. If you are easily awakened by light, you may prefer a clock with a flashing light. If you are a deep sleeper, consider the vibrating unit mentioned above, which can be placed under the pillow or mattress. If a gentle breeze is sufficient to wake you up, consider an electric fan connected to a timer.

Smoke or fire alarms. If you are concerned about being able to hear the alarm from your smoke detector, you may want to purchase a smoke detector that combines a built-in horn and a strobe light. Others have a separate horn that plugs into an electrical outlet in the bedroom or elsewhere in the house. A lamp, strobe, or vibrating device also can plug into a portable receiver.

Hearing the telephone and the doorbell. If you have turned up the telephone ringer volume as high as possible and still can't hear it when the water is running or the television is on, consider a light or vibrating alert. If you cannot hear the doorbell ring when you are a distance from its source, consider placing a ringer in the room you are in most frequently or connecting it to an alerting device.

Paging systems. Battery powered receivers worn on the wrist or the waist can keep you in touch with family and friends. Pagers can receive messages from touch-tone phones, personal computers, and TTYs. Vibrating pagers with alphanumeric display screens offer a new way to contact hard of hearing people.

In the car. If you are not able to hear sirens or your turn signal when driving, you could be placing yourself in a dangerous situation unnecessarily. Two signaling devices can help you: The emergency response indicator is a signaling device for the automobile that turns on a light when emergency vehicles such as fire, police, or ambulance sirens or car horns are nearby. A turn signal reminder can alert you that your left-right signal is on. Several automobile companies offer a rebate for the complete cost of these devices to hard of hearing people who have purchased their product after 1994.

Hearing Dogs

Hearing dogs are trained by professionals to alert their owners to various significant sounds. When one of these sounds occurs, the dog attracts the owner's attention and leads him or her to the sound. In the case of a fire alarm, the dog attracts the owner's attention and then drops to the ground. Hearing dogs may be any breed or mixed breed. They are working animals and can be reliable protectors and loving, loyal companions. Like all dogs, they must be fed, kept clean, walked, and loved. Hearing dogs are permitted in all public places, just as are seeing-eye dogs for people with vision loss. If you live alone, you may wish to consider owning a hearing dog (see Appendix B).

Purchasing Signaling Devices

The number of signaling and alerting devices on the market grows daily and making a decision about the best one to buy is not easy. Your audiologist can provide guidance. Visit a hearing rehabilitation center if one is located near you. Talk to other hard of hearing people who have purchased devices and have found them helpful. The best place to try out a variety of devices is at the annual convention of Self Help for Hard of Hearing People, Inc. For a list of the several demonstration centers in the United States, contact Self Help for Hard of Hearing People (see Appendix B).

19

HEARING ON
THE TELEPHONE

So much of our lives revolves around using the telephone—it is our connection with the world. We use it to make appointments, chat with family and friends, and call for help in an emergency. We need to use the telephone if we are in the work force and also if we are community volunteers. Good telephone communication has long been a requirement for hard of hearing individuals.

Some people with hearing loss hear well on the telephone, but many people with hearing loss need to have the sound amplified moderately. Others need to use a hearing aid with a telecoil (T-switch) to receive the message clearly, while still others may need to use a TTY or other telephone device.

The T-switch
The T-switch, variously known as the telecoil, the induction coil, and the induction pick-up coil, is the term used to describe a special feature on a hearing aid that uses the principle of inductive coupling. The T-switch has many uses besides telephone communication since it can link the hearing aid to other sources of electromagnetic energy, the most common of which are the audioloop system and a host of assistive listening devices (see Key 17).

Hard of hearing people have found that hearing aids with telecoils can be used with much success on telephones that are hearing-aid compatible. Flipping a small switch from the normal setting to the "T" setting when using a hearing aid on the telephone not only reduces the sound of background noise but makes it easier to concentrate on the conversation. If your hearing aid does not have a telecoil, you may want to explore having a telecoil added or consider an aid with a telecoil when you purchase a new one.

Telephone Devices
You may wish to investigate the many telephone listening devices on the market that meet the varying needs of hard of hearing people. Some people find older, reconditioned telephones provide the best reception.

Choosing the right telephone device depends on your needs and the environment in which you will use it. Before buying any device, try different kinds of equipment. Ask other people with hearing loss about their experience with the product. Each device has advantages and disadvantages. Consider your needs along with the cost of the device.

Amplified telephones. Telephones can be amplified by using a handset with a volume control built in, a portable amplifier that slips onto the handset, or an in-line amplifier attached to a regular phone. Amplifiers can be used with or without a hearing aid.

1. **Built-in amplifiers.** If you regularly use the same telephone, you can replace the standard handset with one that has a built-in amplifier. The volume control allows you to set the volume at a comfortable level and also allows you to adjust the volume for different voices. Other people using the same handset can adjust the level to the normal volume. When replacing the standard handset with an amplified one, be sure it will function with the brand and model of the telephone.
2. **Portable amplifiers.** These are convenient when traveling or if you use several different telephones. With this device, the battery-powered amplifier slips over the handset earpiece, and you can adjust the volume to suit your needs. Although easy to attach and operate,

the portable amplifier may not work on all telephones or make the volume as loud as some hard of hearing people need it to be.

3. **In-line amplifiers.** These are connected between the base of the telephone and the standard handset and are best for a permanent placement. The device allows you to adjust the volume as needed. Before you buy one, make sure it will function with the brand and model of the telephone to which you intend to connect it.

TTYs. If you find that neither amplification nor the T-switch allow you to communicate well on the telephone, consider a TTY, sometimes called a TT or TDD. TTYs make it possible for hard of hearing people who cannot use an amplified telephone to communicate over a standard telephone. TTYs are made up of a typewriter-like keyboard, a telephone coupler, and some form of visual display. The visual display may be in the form of printed characters on paper, an alphanumeric display, or both. To use a TTY, you place the telephone handset on the coupler and type the message you wish to send. When you press characters on the keyboard to type in the message, a series of tones is generated. There is a different set of tones for each character. Those tones that form the typed message are sent over the telephone lines to the telephone on the other end of the line. This telephone also must be linked to a TTY so that the message can be decoded and displayed. The latest models of TTYs have a voice carry-over (VCO) mode so that the hard of hearing person can speak the message but receive the answer on the TTY.

Telecommunications relay services. Another option for hard of hearing people is the telecommunications relay service, which acts as an intermediary between a TTY user and a person speaking on a regular voice telephone. To use a relay service, you dial the number on the TTY. The specially trained relay operator on duty reads your typed message and relays the information to the person on another telephone. The operator then types the spoken reply back to you via the TTY. You may want to use voice carry-over mode with the relay service as well. In a VCO call, you speak directly to the other party, whose voiced response is typed back to you by the relay operator. TTYs are often available free or at reduced rates through your state relay program. Since 1993 relay services are available in all 50 states for calls placed within the state and throughout the world.

Electronic mail. The computer age has ushered in another popular way to communicate, e-mail. Although you may not own a computer with an electronic mail program, and not everyone you want to communicate with has a computer with a program, this option is becoming increasingly popular.

Telephone answering machines. You may find that trying to understand the message on your answering machine is frustrating. Manufacturers are developing machines with an audio output jack. When the jack is used, the internal loudspeaker is bypassed. Hard of hearing people can use the answering machine by either plugging in high-quality headphones or using a neckloop to inductively couple the output to the hearing aid telecoil.

Caller I.D. Most telephone companies offer Caller I.D., which lets you see the name and number of the incoming call before you answer the telephone. Knowing who you are talking to before picking up the receiver often helps you get over the initial embarrassment of not getting a caller's name.

Cellular phones. Cellular telephones have become increasingly popular. They are exempt from federal legislation that ensures that phones are accessible to people with hearing loss; however, most of them have volume control and some have built-in hearing aid compatibility (HAC). If you purchase a cellular telephone, be sure you try different models to determine which sounds best and is easiest to use.

Digital wireless telephones. A new generation of cellular telephone, called a digital wireless telephone, recently was introduced into some communities in the United States. These new phones have many advantages, such as the ability to link with computers and fax machines and a clarity of sound not often found with other wireless telephones. Unfortunately, hearing aid wearers may experience a buzzing sound due to the interference these telephones cause when they are in close proximity to some hearing aids and other hearing technology. Several consumer organizations, including Self Help for Hard of Hearing People, are working with equipment providers and hearing aid manufacturers to address these problems. It is difficult to predict which aids and which telephones will be immune to interference; therefore, you must use trial and error when selecting a digital phone.

Hearing the Telephone Ring

If you have difficulty hearing the telephone ring, an amplified telephone ringer can help. If you set it at the greatest volume and this is not sufficient, you may want to install a device that flashes a light when the phone rings (see Key 18). Some ringers are designed for easy listening by producing a lower tone.

20

COCHLEAR IMPLANTS

If you have a severe to profound hearing loss and have received minimal benefit from hearing aids because of the severity of your loss, you may wish to explore the benefits of a cochlear implant. A cochlear implant is a device that is partially implanted into the bone behind the ear to stimulate remaining nerve fibers within the inner ear. The device helps most recipients hear environmental sounds, helps improve speechreading, helps monitor their own speech, and often helps recipients understand voices without looking at the speaker. Some people even report that they can enjoy the sound of music again. It is not unusual for implant recipients to have full use of the telephone.

A cochlear implant is not a cure nor does it restore hearing to normal. It is an example of advanced technology that taps the retained potential of the hearing pathway even in profound deafness by enabling it to respond to sound by bypassing damaged hair cells to directly activate auditory nerve fibers. Many recipients say they function as well as people who have been effectively fitted with hearing aids.

How They Work

The cochlear implant works as follows: Sound waves enter the implant through the microphone located in an earpiece and are converted into an electrical signal. The signal is sent to the wearable speech processor, which transforms each sound into a distinctive code. Because speech sounds have their own distinctive "fingerprint" of energy peaks, they can be differentiated by the cochlear implant. Signals are then sent back and transmitted through the skin via radio waves to the implanted cochlear stimulator. The stimulator, in turn, decodes the received signal and delivers it to the implanted electrode contact. The contact stimulates the nerve endings within the cochlea, which convey impulses to the brain where they are interpreted as sound.

The ideal candidate for a cochlear implant has a severe to profound sensorineural hearing loss in both ears, has tried hearing aids with little or no success, and has no medical conditions that contraindicate the surgery. These medical contraindications are quite rare but include conditions that make a general anesthetic risky, such as severe coronary artery disease, a chronic pulmonary condition, or a genetic condition that interferes with the metabolism of anesthetic agents.

Success depends on the ability to acclimate to a new format of speech sounds provided by the implant. Patient motivation, the length of time the patient has had a hearing loss, and an extensive memory of sound and language are important factors that predict high levels of performance in understanding speech with a cochlear implant.

Cochlear implants have been in use for 25 years and have improved dramatically during the last five years. The Food and Drug Administration has approved two devices for use with adults, and, in 1990, approved them for children.

If you are interested in exploring your candidacy for a cochlear implant, you will need several tests, some of which are the same as those you would have if you were assessing the potential benefits of a hearing aid. A hearing test and a hearing aid evaluation are initially performed (see Key 11). You also will need a medical and psychological evaluation to assess your medical suitability, level of motivation, and expectations. Other tests that help predict success of the procedure provide the implant team with needed information to determine which ear to implant via electrical stimulation of the auditory nerve.

The Actual Surgery

The surgery, performed under general anesthesia, is relatively pain free, takes two to three hours, and complications are rare. Implant recipients leave the hospital within 24 to 48 hours, although the surgery is performed increasingly as an outpatient procedure.

The surgeon makes an incision behind the ear, raises a skin flap to expose part of the mastoid bone, and drills a small depression in the bone to hold the receiver/stimulator (internal coil) in place. The cochlear implant is placed under the skin with stimulating arrays consisting of electrical contacts threaded into the cochlea. The array of contacts is inserted into the cochlea through a small opening near the round window. The skin flap is sutured; healing takes about four weeks.

All cochlear implants have internal and external parts. The internal parts—internal coil and electrodes—are inserted during surgery. The external parts—microphone, speech processor, and external antenna—are hooked together and linked via magnet to the internal parts after the incision has healed. At this time, the audiologist assesses the patient's ability to listen for sounds and adjusts controls in the speech processor. The speech processor is the size of a small calculator, and is worn externally as the speech decoder that drives the implant. The assessment may take several visits since the patient needs to adapt to new sounds that initially are different from the sounds heard through a hearing aid. With experience, many implant recipients note enhanced fidelity or sound quality.

Cost

Cochlear implants are expensive and currently cost from $20,000 to $30,000. This includes the evaluation, surgery, hospital costs, fitting the device, and communication training. Many health insurance carriers, including Medicare in most states, provide full or partial coverage for cochlear implant devices.

If you think you might be a candidate for a cochlear implant, talk to an otolaryngologist who may refer you to a specialist in this field. For a list of qualified specialists, contact:

The American Academy of Otolaryngology—Head
   and Neck Surgery, Inc.
One Prince Street
Alexandria, Virginia 22314
(703) 836-4444

21

SPEECHREADING

Many people with hearing loss use their eyes to make up for what they cannot hear since they usually have difficulty hearing speech as it normally sounds. You may have noticed that in addition to straining to hear what is being said, you also are using your eyes to get what your ears miss and that you seem to hear better when you see people's faces.

In the normal course of interacting with others, we all develop some degree of speechreading skill. Some of this skill involves lipreading, the recognizing of sounds by shapes and movements of the speaker's mouth. Lipreading, however, is difficult because only 30 to 40 percent of speech is visible on the lips. Many sounds are made in the back of the throat, such as *k* and hard *g*. Also, many words have the same mouth movement and look the same on the lips, but sound different, such as *pat*, *bat*, and *mat*. Speechreading can be a little bit like taking a fill-in-the-blanks test, so paying attention to context is critical to good speechreading.

Your friends and family will often say, "You speechread, don't you?" Yes, you do, but you need to let them know that not all hard of hearing people read speech as easily and accurately as hearing people can listen to it, and not all hard of hearing people are skilled at speechreading. It is a skill that must be learned and practiced regularly. Some hard of hearing people are more successful than others because they hear better, and some simply have a special talent for speechreading.

When you speechread, it does not mean that you ignore your hearing; even a little bit of residual hearing can enhance speechreading ability. As it turns out, the sounds that are hardest to differentiate visually, like *p*, *b*, and *m*—because they are formed the same way on the lips—are the easiest ones to perceive through hearing. Conversely, the sounds that are likely to be the hardest to hear, like *s*, *f*, and *th* are the easiest ones to see. Good speechreaders combine all they can see and all they can hear for the purpose of improving speech comprehension.

People who have a regional accent, speak a language other than English, do not use much mouth movement, or have a mustache are more difficult to speechread. Unfamiliar topics and vocabulary as well as sudden changes of topic also can cause problems for the hard of hearing person. You will be able to improve your comprehension once you are familiar with the topic being discussed. You also may become better able to speechread individuals once you become accustomed to the way they speak.

Speechreading, like any new skill, is more likely to be acquired if you receive training, practice regularly, and have natural ability. Receiving encouragement from others helps, too. Unfortunately, classes are hard to find and are also usually short-term (eight to ten weeks), which is only a beginning. So you will have to work out a disciplined approach on your own. Try asking a relative or friend to work regularly with you, or seek out a local group that is also interested in speechreading, perhaps at a community center, senior center, place of worship, or SHHH group.

Speechreading videotapes and guidebooks are available, and some community colleges offer classes to help people refine their skills. Many of the chapters of Self Help for Hard of Hearing People offer speechreading courses.

22

WILL AN ORAL
INTERPRETER HELP?

If you depend on speechreading to get information, you probably have no trouble participating and following the flow of conversation in one-to-one and small group situations. However, when there is audience participation or when the speaker is on the stage or some distance away, you may find speechreading difficult, if not impossible.

You may understand the speaker by sitting close and using assistive devices; audioloops or infrared systems also may help, when available. When neither of these is helpful, you might consider engaging an oral interpreter.

Well-meaning people may offer suggestions about using sign language interpreters to help you understand in large group situations, but learning sign language takes a great deal of patience and many years of practice. An oral interpreter, however, might provide the support you need in certain situations.

What Is an Oral Interpreter?
Oral interpreters sit near you and repeat silently what is said at the time it is spoken, following two or three words behind the speaker. They simultaneously convey the mood and meaning of the message with expression and natural gestures. Oral interpreters are trained to mouth distinctly, may substitute a word that is easier to speechread, and may rephrase, all for the purpose of producing clear speech. If asked, the oral interpreters will use their voice to repeat the message if the speaker has unclear speech, a foreign accent, or wears a mustache or beard that might make speechreading difficult.

When to Consider Using an Oral Interpreter

If you are frustrated in meetings, seminars, and other situations in which you are not able to hear clearly, you may wish to consider using an oral interpreter. An oral interpreter is most helpful when the speaker is on the telephone or radio, providing narration that accompanies a TV or other audiovisual presentation, or has a foreign or regional accent. If you are unable to sit close to the speaker or if several people are speaking at the same time, using an oral interpreter can help your comprehension. Remember, however, that unless you are a skilled speechreader, you will not receive the entire message.

Many hard of hearing people who use residual hearing and speechreading to understand the speaker usually are not satisfied users of oral interpreters since the oral interpreter is several words behind the speaker.

How to Find an Oral Interpreter

If an interpreting service is not listed in your telephone book, you can contact the Registry of Interpreters for the Deaf (RID) for suggestions (see Appendix B). Interpreters are professionals who graduate with a minimum of two years of training at a college or university and are certified or state approved based on written and performance evaluations. They are paid on an hourly basis. Fees vary from state to state.

It is your responsibility to pay for the interpreter if the service you need is personal, such as in a social situation. Under the Americans with Disabilities Act (ADA) (see Key 28), if you need an interpreter to participate in a program or service, the public accommodation, state or local government facility, or place of employment should pay the fee. For example, if you need an interpreter to understand hospital medical staff, the hospital should provide a qualified interpreter at no cost to you.

23

ASSERTIVE COMMUNICATION

Being Assertive

As a hard of hearing person, you may experience anger and frustration while trying to understand and be understood. You can cope with some of these communication frustrations you experience daily by learning simple assertiveness techniques.

Don't let the word assertive or the concept of assertive behavior scare you. There is a difference between *assertive* behavior and *aggressive* behavior. Assertiveness is a positive attribute. If you use assertive techniques, you will find that you can make things happen, change people's behavior, and, what is more important, change your own behavior. Aggressive behavior, on the other hand, is a negative approach and usually has negative results.

The following example will illustrate how you can communicate the same message in several ways, as well as the importance of communicating assertively.

You and your hearing companion arrive at a hotel and prepare to register. The desk clerk hands you a card and pen. You fill out the card, and, as you wait for your room key, the desk clerk with head down asks for your credit card. You know the clerk is saying something, but you do not understand him and cannot see his face. How do you react?

1. You smile sweetly and act as if you didn't hear anything.
2. You ask your companion to tell you what the clerk said.
3. You angrily say something like, "Look at me when you speak to me, and speak louder!"

4. You calmly say, "I am hard of hearing. It will help me to hear you if you look at me when you speak."

Reactions 1 and 2 are examples of *passive behavior*, acting as if you understand what is going on when you don't. This behavior is often accompanied by a "sweet smile," a vague expression, letting someone else be your ears, and not letting other people know that you are hard of hearing. Passive behavior keeps you from dealing with the reality of your hearing loss. It makes you dependent on others. It often causes others to ignore you and to think of you as less capable than you are.

Reaction 3 is called *aggressive behavior*. Examples of aggressive behavior are acting as if you are right and the world is wrong, demanding rather than asking for support, blaming others when you don't understand, dominating the conversation, and insisting on hearing everything. Hard of hearing people often use aggressive behavior to hide their disability. It does not solve communication problems; rather, it lowers self-esteem and may cause resentment in others, who may do what you ask but then may avoid interacting with you in the future.

Reaction 4 is an example of *assertive behavior*. Acting for yourself, accepting your hearing loss, taking responsibility for your actions, and communicating clearly to let others know what they can do to be helpful are elements of assertive behavior.

Assertive behavior allows you to act in your own best interests, to stand up for yourself, to express your feelings comfortably, and to exercise your rights while not infringing on the rights of others. With assertive behavior, you say: "I know I have a problem. I am asking for your help, and I am telling you what I need."

Assertive behavior is not easy. It takes much practice, but after a while, what you say and what you do becomes second nature.

Body Language

Assertiveness is not only verbal, meaning what you say and how you say it. Many other nonverbal factors—known as body language—come into play, including:

- eye contact
- body posture
- distance/physical contact
- gestures
- facial expressions
- voice tone, inflection, and volume
- pace of speech
- timing

Body language can send a very different message than the words you are saying. When your body says one thing and your voice says another, the body language prevails.

Taking Responsibility

Remember your hearing problem is just that—*your* problem. It is not anyone else's problem. It is your responsibility to take charge of the situation and help yourself and, at the same time, not make others feel uncomfortable. When you have recognized and accepted that you have a hearing loss, have had your hearing tested and evaluated, and have purchased hearing aids, you have already taken a large measure of responsibility (see Key 24).

Being assertive can make a big difference in your life. You can become more assertive by saying what is on your mind, expressing yourself honestly, and respecting your rights and the rights of others. Getting what you want and what you need is not always easy. Getting what you need and not infringing on the rights of others is an art.

If you want to learn more about assertive techniques that will help you deal with your hearing loss and with other general situations, you will find books and videos on this subject in your library. Courses on assertiveness are often taught at community colleges and offered by many SHHH chapters.

24

TIPS FOR IMPROVING COMMUNICATION

Once friends, relatives, and others with whom you interact are aware that you have a hearing loss, they will want to know how best to communicate with you. Being specific about your needs will provide an opportunity for you to help others while helping yourself. Don't just say "I have a hearing loss." Tell people exactly what they can do to help.

You are the primary decision maker when choosing the appropriate environment for communication. You need to tell people with whom you are talking that you can't hear well when the water is running, the television is on, their back is turned, when others in the room are carrying on an animated conversation, and in any situation that causes a problem for you. A quiet place with no background noise is priority number one. Lighting is important, too; it should be on the speaker's face in order for you to receive maximum benefit. Since sound disperses with distance, you should get as close as you can to the speaker. If appropriate, encourage the speaker to use facial expressions and gestures.

Below are a few tips for improving communication that you can use to educate other people and take control of your life. Ask them to do the following:

- **Please get my attention before speaking to me.** Ask the speaker to tap you on the shoulder, wave, or use another gesture before beginning to speak.
- **Please give me a clue.** Knowing what the topic of conversation is can help you understand better. Ask the

speaker to say something such as "Lunch. Where shall we have lunch?"

- **Please face me.** Asking the speaker to look at you when talking helps you to hear and speechread more effectively. Position yourself so that the speaker's face is not in the shadows.
- **Please speak slowly and clearly.** Explain that the speaker need not shout nor exaggerate speech. Exaggeration and overemphasis of words distort lip movements, making speechreading more difficult.
- **Please rephrase rather than repeat.** If you do not understand the first time, ask the speaker to rephrase the sentence. You may only miss one or two words, and repetition may help you understand the message the second time around. However, rephrasing often is a better solution.
- **Please talk directly to me.** If you find that people often talk to your hearing companion or spouse when they should be talking to you, be assertive and ask that they talk directly to you. You may need to coach them, but your efforts will pay off with positive results and the communication you need.
- **Please don't cover your mouth when talking to me.** People often talk when eating, chewing on a pencil, or in some way obscuring their mouth. Let them know that this makes speechreading difficult.
- **Please turn off the television or radio.** Background noise is one main reason for not hearing well. Help yourself by requesting that noise be turned down or off before engaging in conversation. You might also suggest moving to a quieter spot.
- **Please don't shout.** Shouting makes things worse. It distorts the face and mouth of the speaker, often making speechreading impossible. If you wear a hearing aid, shouting causes increased vibrations and distorts sound.

In addition to helping other people learn what they can do to facilitate communication, you can do the following:

- **Pay attention.** You need to watch, listen, and concentrate to follow conversation. Daydreaming cuts off communication.
- **Concentrate on the speaker.** If the conversation is important, pay close attention to the speaker. You become a better conversationalist because you focus on one person at a time and are not disturbed by other people and events.
- **Look for visual cues.** Watch for facial expressions, gestures, and body language, which are signs that indicate if conversation is proceeding well.
- **Ask for written cues if needed.** Always carry a notepad and pencil. If you are really stuck, ask the speaker to write key word(s) for you. Sometimes a key word will put the conversation back on track.
- **Don't interrupt. Let conversation flow awhile to gain more meaning.** Sometimes you pick up the missed key word a few sentences later so that what is being discussed makes sense. Give the interchange a chance before you interrupt, but if you are lost, explain and ask for repetition or rephrasing.

Note: One way to ensure that good communication continues is to provide feedback. Let others know what they are doing right. Also, let them know what could be done differently in order to enhance communication. Saying "Thank you" is the best way to provide positive feedback.

25

REARRANGING YOUR HOME ENVIRONMENT

In your own home you can make several changes that make hearing and understanding speech easier. Arrange the furniture where you most frequently sit and converse so that you are close to the person or persons with whom you talk. Position your chair so that your back is to the light source and the light from a window or lamp is on the other person's face. Consider installing better lighting if yours is recessed, since this type of lighting creates shadows and makes speechreading difficult.

You may wish to arrange your chair so that you are able to see people entering a room. This will prevent you from being startled if you can't hear someone come in and frightened if you are tapped on the shoulder from behind.

Background and other noise is often disturbing, so when conversing, turn the television, radio, or stereo down or off. If you are in someone else's home or office, don't be afraid to explain that you will hear better if there is no background noise. Noise reverberation also makes hearing and understanding difficult. Consider dampening reverberation with sound-absorbing material such as carpeting, draperies, and upholstered furniture.

If you can hear better in one ear than the other, position the speaker close to the better ear. Remember to do this when you are in a restaurant or at the theater, also.

If you have difficulty understanding the voices on television, consider purchasing a TV listening device that will enable you to hear without turning the volume too loud for other listeners (see Key 17).

If you have trouble understanding on the telephone, investigate the many telephone devices on the market that meet the varying needs of hard of hearing people. Choosing the right device depends on your needs and the environment in which you will use it (see Key 19).

If you have trouble hearing the telephone ring or someone knocking on your door, consider installing visual signaling devices to compensate for your hearing loss that at the same time allow you to gain a greater sense of awareness. Visual signaling devices—some very inexpensive, others more elaborate—will provide visual alerts such as flashing lights, or vibrations, to indicate the source of a sound such as timers on ovens, a washing machine cycle ending, and other household sounds that help you in your daily work around the house. A visual smoke detector is another device that will provide a sense of confidence and security at home (see Key 18).

You may even consider remodeling. If so, contemplate an open-space design, which is better than closed rooms, since it allows you to visually keep track of what is going on in all parts of your living area.

If you need glasses, wear them. You use your eyes more than ever when you lose your hearing. Your sense of sight becomes more critical in order to compensate for what you don't hear. If low vision is reducing your ability to cope with hearing loss and communicate effectively, you need to make adjustments in many areas. A dual sensory loss requires learning how to use whatever hearing and vision remain, together with some additional strategies (see Key 24).

26

LIVING ALONE

People with hearing loss must face a number of challenges and responsibilities in order to live alone and function independently: using the telephone; hearing the doorbell and wake-up alarm; enjoying television, radio, and stereo; and dealing with health care, repairs, and other service providers. How can you remain in control of your life and your decisions?

1. You can enjoy an independent and relaxed lifestyle by acknowledging your hearing loss.
2. If you use a hearing aid, wear it every day—not only for special occasions.
3. Learn about the many assistive devices that can be used in concert with hearing aids.
4. Consider refining your speechreading skills.
5. Learn techniques for modifying and controlling your living and social environments.
6. Let other people know that you have a hearing loss and explain your communication needs clearly.

By discovering new ways to adapt you can participate fully in the world around you.

If you are one of the 22.6 percent of people with a hearing loss who live alone, the following strategies might help you learn how to remain independent.

- **Hearing the telephone and the doorbell.** A variety of alerting devices and systems that use a flashing light or vibrations are available to alert you to door knocks, doorbells, telephones, burglar alarms, smoke and fire alarms, and other sounds you may have difficulty hearing.
- **Hearing on the telephone.** Telephone listening devices can increase the loudness of sound coming through the

telephone. They can be used with or without a hearing aid. If you have difficulty hearing on the telephone, a telephone with built-in volume control or an amplified handset might be the solution. You may want to try a portable amplifier when you are away from your home phone. If your hearing loss is more profound, consider using a TTY as well as telecommunications relay services.

- **Waking up at a specified time.** Specialized wake-up alarms for hard of hearing people include digital and standard clocks, bed vibrators, and timers. Clocks that use a flashing light for the alarm are useful for people easily awakened by light. For heavy sleepers, several kinds of bed-vibrating units may be helpful. Some can be placed under a pillow or mattress. Some are small enough for travel. Timers or clocks with built-in electrical outlets allow you to choose whether to use a light or vibrator.

- **Listening to television, radio, and stereo.** TV, radio, and stereo listening devices allow you to increase the loudness of sound without disturbing other people or damaging your residual hearing. Some devices can be connected to the TV, radio, or stereo when using an audio input hearing aid, by using earphones instead of a hearing aid, or by using an induction loop. A TV caption decoder allows the viewer to see text of TV dialogue of programs that are captioned. All TV sets that are 13 inches and larger, manufactured after July 1, 1993, have a built-in chip that allows users to see captions without a decoder (see Key 17).

- **Receiving emergency warnings.** Many hard of hearing people worry about not hearing the alarm from their smoke detectors. Some smoke detectors combine a built-in horn and a strobe light; others have a separate horn that plugs into an electrical outlet in the bedroom or elsewhere in the house. A lamp, strobe, or vibrating device also can plug into a portable receiver. Emergency alarm devices can automatically call the fire department and give the person's address when a smoke detector goes off. Other emergency alarm devices call an emergency service (police, fire, or ambulance) and play a recorded message at the press of a button (see Key 19).

Problems Away from Home

- **In the hospital.** Hospitalization, while often stressful for many, can be even more disturbing for a hard of hearing person whose anxieties are compounded by the fear of not hearing or understanding questions and instructions, announcements, and directions. While all patients in hospitals need advocates, your needs as a hard of hearing patient are even more critical (see Key 32).
- **While traveling.** If you need and want to travel alone for business or personal enjoyment, you can continue to remain independent and effective by careful planning and exercising special techniques (see Key 33).
- **At the hairdresser/barber.** Difficulty communicating while having your hair washed, cut, and styled can be overcome with a little effort. By alerting the hairdresser/barber that decisions must be made and discussion held before you remove your hearing aid(s), you will be using specialized communication techniques and educating others at the same time.

Hearing Dogs

You may wish to consider a hearing dog that is trained to respond to sounds and alert you to them (see Key 18).

A Final Word of Advice

Try various devices and systems and evaluate them to find what works best for your level of hearing loss with and without a hearing aid. Also, learn special communication techniques that allow you to remain independent. Remember that many hard of hearing people are living alone successfully, and so can you.

27

THE INTERNATIONAL SYMBOL OF ACCESS FOR HEARING LOSS

You have a new friend: The International Symbol of Access for Hearing Loss. Used worldwide, this symbol identifies locations where communication access is provided.

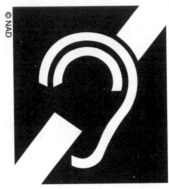

Figure 4 The International Symbol of Access for Hearing Loss.

The symbol (Figure 4) is typically white with a blue background. You will see it on public phones and know that they are hearing-aid compatible and have amplification. You will see it posted outside meeting rooms and in places of entertainment and worship to indicate that the room is equipped with an assistive listening system. You will see it posted on patients' doors in hospitals to alert hospital personnel to the fact that the patient has a hearing loss.

Wherever you see it, you will know that people are aware of hearing loss and have responded by providing communication accessibility.

28

WHAT ARE
YOUR LEGAL RIGHTS?
THE ADA

In the past, many older Americans experienced age discrimination in the workplace. They were passed over during hiring and often for promotion. When they also had a hearing loss, they may have experienced double discrimination. Because of recent legislation, this discrimination is occurring less frequently. Still, many people with disabilities, including those with hearing loss, are unaware of the several laws that protect their civil rights. Others are reluctant to ask for accommodations that would help them participate in everyday activities. The Americans with Disabilities Act (ADA) (Public Law 101-336) is comprehensive federal legislation affirming the rights of persons with disabilities to equal access.

The Americans with Disabilities Act
The ADA, enacted in 1990 to protect people with physical or mental disabilities, ensures that all Americans have access to employment (Title I), public services and public transportation (Title II), public accommodations (Title III), and telecommunications (Title IV). The ADA states that no individual may be discriminated against on the basis of disability in the "full and equal enjoyment" of the services or facilities of any place of "public accommodation." Because hearing loss is considered a disability, you are protected under the law.

If you are employed or seeking employment, the ADA guarantees you equal opportunity. Employers must reasonably accommodate the disabilities of qualified applicants or current employees, unless an undue hardship would result.

You should have access to all local, state, and federal government facilities, services, and communication. Public buses and bus stations, and trains and train stations, need to comply with the ADA. Airlines are covered by the Air Carriers Access Act, but airports must provide accessibility under the ADA.

You should have access to public accommodations. This means that hotels, restaurants, theaters, retail stores, museums, libraries, and parks must include services that make it easier for you to hear. Hospitals, pharmacies, and doctors' offices also must comply. Places of worship and private clubs are exempt from the ADA; many of these, however, provide access for people with hearing loss.

Telephone companies must provide free relay service to people with hearing loss who use TTYs or similar devices 24 hours a day, seven days a week.

If You Believe that You Have Been Discriminated Against

If you believe that you have been discriminated against, you have several options. Assuming you have exhausted all methods of negotiation with your employer, facility manager, etc., it is a good idea to first try mediation. This can be done through local mediation centers, conflict resolution services, and legal offices specializing in disputes. This strategy has proved successful in avoiding litigation. If mediation fails, you have the following legal recourse:

In employment: You may file a complaint with the Equal Employment Opportunity Commission (EEOC).

In public accommodations: You can bring a private lawsuit to obtain court orders to stop discrimination, but money damages cannot be awarded. Or you can file a complaint with the U.S. Attorney General, who may file lawsuits to stop discrimination and obtain money damages and penalties.

In transportation: You may file a complaint with the U.S. Department of Transportation or bring a private lawsuit.

In state and local government operations: You may file a complaint with federal agencies to be designated by the U.S. Attorney General or bring a private lawsuit.

In telecommunications: You may file a complaint with the Federal Communications Commission (FCC).

Other Relevant Legislation
The Hearing Aid Compatibility Act of 1988 stipulates that all telephones manufactured in the United States or imported for use in the United States must provide internal means for effective use with hearing aids that are designed to be compatible with telephones that meet established technical standards for hearing aid compatibility.

TV Decoder Circuitry Act of 1990 stipulates that all televisions with screens 13 inches and larger manufactured since 1993 must contain a built-in decoder chip.

The Rehabilitation Act of 1973 states that all people have a right to equal opportunities. Title V of the act specifies that facilities and programs receiving federal funds be accessible to all disabled persons. Under section 502 of Title V, buildings and facilities that are designed, constructed, altered, or leased with federal funds must be communication accessible. Section 504 of the act deals with federally funded programs and activities. The act prohibits discrimination against people with disabilities such as employees, participants, or viewers.

29

HEARING IN RESTAURANTS

Many social and business activities take place at mealtimes and in restaurants. It is difficult for most people to watch their food and the face of their companion(s) simultaneously, but for people with hearing loss, it can cause greater problems and significant frustration.

If your dining companion is a close relative or friend whose voice you are used to, and the subject matter you will be discussing is familiar, you may have no problem hearing. If, however, the meal is for business purposes, with someone you have met recently, with a larger group, or with someone who also has a hearing loss, you will communicate more successfully by taking a number of factors into account when choosing a restaurant. These include noise level, lighting, and seating.

Most people choose restaurants for the quality and variety of food, and the service, ambiance, and price. Hard of hearing people need to take other things into consideration when dining out in order to increase their ability to understand conversation.

Below are a few suggestions for making your restaurant dining experience more enjoyable.

- Call ahead, if possible. Tell the person accepting the reservation that you are hard of hearing and would like a table in a quiet spot. You may need to explain that "quiet" means little or no noise from behind, not near the air conditioning/heating unit or loudspeaker, and certainly not in the center of the room. A corner table or a booth in the back is often a good choice.

- Timing is important. The best times for lower noise levels are before and after peak hours. Not only are restaurants crowded at noon and 6:30 P.M., but service is usually rushed.
- Choose a restaurant with good lighting. Some restaurants have low levels of lighting, which can make it difficult to speechread and see facial expressions. Music often accompanies soft lights. Don't hesitate to ask the waiter to turn down or turn off the music if a speaker near you is causing difficulty hearing.
- Choose the seat at the table that will maximize your ability to hear the conversation. If you hear better in one ear than in the other, ask your companion or the person you most wish to hear to sit on the better side. A seat against a wall is a good choice because you will not have sound coming to you from behind. If the restaurant has windows or bright lighting, be sure that your back is to the light so that your companions' faces are not in the shadows.
- Restaurants often offer specials. Ask the waiter if these are written down so that you can read them; if not, ask the waiter to stand closer to you so that you can speechread and hear better.
- If you own an FM system or another one-on-one communicator, be sure to take it with you to facilitate conversation with your dinner companions and the waiter.
- If you are unable to make a reservation beforehand and find yourself in a noisy restaurant or at a noisy table where communication would be difficult, and it is important that you be able to understand what is being said, consider leaving and finding another restaurant.

While most restaurant personnel are helpful and understanding, you need to tell them that you have a hearing loss and what they can do to help you hear. When they provide help, show your gratitude; when they don't, you can make your dissatisfaction known, courteously, but firmly.

Drive-Thrus

For those of you who enjoy fast-food dining, the drive-thru procedure can be challenging since you are unable to see the face of the person taking your order, and the audio system often is poor quality. In order to take advantage of this convenient way to get a meal without leaving your automobile, be prepared to place your order when you hear the "squawk" at the drive-up box. Speak clearly and provide information as completely as possible, ending with the statement "That's all, thank you." Drive on to the payment window, where the order taker will relay any unanswered questions. You may have a delay at the window, but the procedure may be faster than standing in line inside and useful when you are tired or in a hurry.

Bon Appetit!

30

HEARING IN
THEATERS AND MOVIES

If you enjoyed theater productions and movies before you lost your hearing, you will wish to continue to enjoy them now. Since the passage of the Americans with Disabilities Act, most theaters and movie houses (and public facilities in general, including sports arenas) have installed systems designed to accommodate people with hearing loss. One way to ensure that accessibility to movies and theaters continues is to use these systems and let theater owners and managers know if they are working well.

Some theaters advertise in local newspaper movie guides that they have special audio systems in place. Others fail to advertise so you may need to call and inquire if the theater has a system available. The newspaper may also tell what kinds of devices are available. Most theaters have headphones. Some have neckloops for hard of hearing people who have T-switches on their hearing aids.

If you have not been able to inquire about assistive devices beforehand, look for signs indicating that assistive devices are available when you arrive at the theater. The International Symbol of Access for Hearing Loss often lets consumers know that the theater is accessible to people with hearing loss (see Key 27). If no signs are posted, ask about accessibility at the ticket counter.

Even though theaters may be in compliance with the ADA, you and other consumers with hearing loss, who have high expectations for the equipment, may come away dissatisfied. Theater personnel sometimes are uninformed or poorly trained so the information provided may be incorrect or insufficient. Imagine what that is like for a first-time user. As a consumer, it will benefit you to become informed so that you can help educate the theater personnel and thus receive maximum benefit from the equipment.

Headphones
The most often used pieces of equipment in movie theaters are wireless, light, and easy to use headphones designed to receive infrared waves. The earphones are attached to a panel displaying a switch and volume control. A thumbwheel can adjust the volume, which operates only when an infrared emitter, usually mounted above the stage, is in operation. A diode at the base of each earphone receives the wireless radiation of the infrared emitter through a hidden eye that faces the stage as you are seated in the theater. The only precaution is that the eye not be obscured by clothes, hands, a person, or object because this will cut off the reception of sound from the infrared emitter.

In order to borrow a device and ensure that it will be returned, you may have to leave a driver's license or other identification with the employee at the ticket counter. It is illegal for theaters to charge for use of the receivers. When you return the equipment at the end of the performance, be sure to let personnel know how much you appreciate having it available. If it worked well for you, mention that. If it is inadequate or not in working order, let the manager of the theater know that the equipment is not providing adequate support or needs repair. When the theater advertises that it provides accommodation for hard of hearing people, it should do so; therefore, it is not unreasonable to ask for a refund if the system is not working properly and you have to leave. If systems are not used, or if they are not doing the job, then nothing will be done to improve them unless you and others speak up.

Above all, don't let the stigma factor of hearing loss keep you from enjoying movies and theater productions. It may be more comfortable to rent a captioned video and stay at home—and this too is an option—but socializing and sharing with others is an important part of remaining active.

31

HEARING IN PLACES OF WORSHIP

If you have difficulty hearing in your place of worship and are unable to participate fully in the service or meetings, consider talking to your minister, priest, or rabbi about the impact of your hearing loss on your spiritual life.

Explain that the inability to hear religious services, announcements, and at special ceremonies relating to celebrations of life results in a deep sense of deprivation and loss. Emphasize that an improved listening environment could provide accessibility for you and other hard of hearing members of the congregation. This is an opportunity for you to be an advocate for yourself and at the same time act on behalf of others.

If your place of worship does not have an assistive listening system (see Key 17), let your clergy know that even though places of worship are exempt from the Americans with Disabilities Act, more and more congregations are employing the use of these systems to help people who are hard of hearing. Many places of worship have systems that are not being used. There could be several reasons for this: The system is not being advertised so congregants are unaware that it is in place, hard of hearing people do not like to be conspicuous by wearing a device, or, often, the system is inadequate or not functioning properly. For example, FM and infrared systems require continual attention to ensure that receivers are in working order, and audio loop systems may not be powerful enough to meet the needs of worshipers.

The mere presence of an audio system is not enough to include hard of hearing people in the activities of the congregation. Members of the congregation need to be educated about the availability of the system and how to use it. Ushers must be trained to guide worshipers to reserved pews that have been installed with devices and offer instruction for their use. They also need to know what seating provides optimal listening if loop systems are installed. You, as an advocate, should use the systems and encourage others to do the same.

Often a system has been installed in the sanctuary. It is equally important that a system be placed in other locations. Explain that when lecture halls and meeting rooms are not equipped with special devices that make dialogue accessible, you miss out on the comfort and inspiration of a spiritual community.

If your place of worship wants to investigate installing a system, a good place to begin is by asking the administration to survey the congregation to determine how many people would benefit from a system. This survey will determine the number of personal receivers, earphones, earbuds, and neckloops needed. It is important also to survey members who have stopped attending services because they did not hear well.

The system considered for installation by your place of worship should accommodate members of the congregation who wear hearing aids as well as those who do not but would benefit from an assistive listening system.

Your church administration may not know where to buy a system. SHHH, hearing clinics, audiologists, and sound system installers can help identify suppliers. You and other hard of hearing congregants should insist on being present when testing systems before purchase and also during the trial period after one is installed to ensure satisfactory operation, since installers may not be aware of your needs.

32

HEARING IN
THE HOSPITAL

Hospitalization, while often stressful for many, can be even more disturbing to a hard of hearing person whose anxieties are compounded by the fear of not hearing or understanding questions, instructions, and announcements. These concerns are not unfounded. If you have difficulty communicating with hospital staff members, it may cause misunderstandings that can affect your treatment and lead to undesirable consequences. Therefore, as a hard of hearing patient, it is essential that you make every effort to establish good communication with the nurses, doctors, and other members of the health care staff.

Preadmission
Use your preadmission visit to inform the admissions office and other hospital personnel of your hearing loss and discuss your communication needs. The preadmission form may ask if you have a hearing loss; if it does not, you should note your hearing loss on the form anyway. Request materials such as brochures and pamphlets that describe the services and equipment available for people with hearing loss. Some hospitals, for example, provide captioned television, one-on-one communicators, and amplified telephone handsets.

In the Hospital
Once you are settled into your room, begin your effort to establish good communication by making sure that your chart is labeled to alert health care providers that you are

hard of hearing. With your consent, a card or the International Symbol of Access for Hearing Loss should be placed on the door (see Key 27). As the nurses and other members of the hospital staff come to your room to greet you, take the opportunity to discuss with each of them your preferred method of communication. If you use assistive devices other than your hearing aid, such as a one-on-one communicator, captioned TV, amplified telephone, or personal FM system, explain to them how the devices operate.

It is not enough to tell people "I am hard of hearing." Educate them. Tell them how to communicate with you by giving them specific strategies such as "try to get my attention before speaking." You may need to repeat this information because staff members may forget, and you may be communicating with different personnel on different shifts. Be patient and polite, but be persistent.

If you do not understand messages over the intercom, ask that information specific for you be delivered face to face. You might suggest that a note or the access symbol be posted at the nurses' station as a reminder when communicating important general information.

It also is important that you understand what the hospital personnel are telling you about your medical condition. If you don't understand what is being communicated, ask to have the information repeated or provided in writing. If you bluff, you may miss important information. Ask about the medications that are prescribed for you because some medications are ototoxic and may adversely affect your hearing (see Key 8). You may wish to have instructions about medications repeated in order to ensure that you clearly understand dosages, purposes, and procedures—and don't hesitate to ask for written instructions.

In addition, if you wear hearing aids, you or a family member or friend should instruct the personnel about the insertion, care, and use of aids as well as the care and testing of batteries, if you are unable to do this for yourself. Tell the staff that when you remove your hearing aids at night or in the shower, you will not be able to hear. Also, be sure that when you remove your hearing aids, they are placed where they won't be lost or damaged and where you can find them easily.

Before and After Surgery

Surgery presents another challenge for a hard of hearing patient since it is difficult, if not impossible, to understand what is being said when the surgical staff members are wearing masks. Inform your surgeon, and particularly your anesthesiologist, of your hearing loss. You may wish to wear your hearing aid during surgery. This is allowed, depending on the type of surgery and equipment used during the procedure. Discuss this with the anesthesiologist. If it is not possible to wear your hearing aid in the operating room, wear it up to the last minute and have a zip-lock bag handy for the aid that is well labeled with your name and room number. You may request that surgical personnel communicate information and instructions before covering their lips.

In the recovery room following surgery, you may encounter personnel who are not aware of your hearing loss. As the anesthesia wears off, you will want to have someone with you who knows how best to communicate with you. Arrange this ahead of time.

As an Outpatient

When you have medical procedures performed in diagnostic laboratories or X-ray departments as an outpatient, you can make the experience less stressful by taking the following steps:

• Tell the receptionist your name and explain that you are hard of hearing.

- Because you may not hear your name when called, ask that someone approach you to get your attention.
- Ask to have "Hard of Hearing" shown prominently on all your medical records as a reminder to the various staff members who interact with you.
- Express your appreciation for the attention you have received.

In the Emergency Room
There are times when you may be unable to prepare for a hospital stay, such as in the event of an accident or sudden illness. It is important for you to plan for hospital emergencies since hearing loss can pose special challenges and risks for you and for the person providing emergency care. Quick recognition that you are hard of hearing is important so that staff members can provide adequate and appropriate care. Keep a card in your wallet that indicates you have a hearing loss and whether you communicate through speechreading or use an assistive device. Remind family members who may accompany you for emergency admission to alert the staff about your hearing loss and how the staff can best communicate with you.

During an emergency, if you are unable to hear because your hearing aid has been damaged or is not working, you may wish to ask for a voice amplifier (a one-on-one communicator). Emergency room personnel may not know that people who are hard of hearing need amplification to communicate rather than a sign language interpreter. However, some hard of hearing patients may need the services of an oral interpreter (see Key 22). Some hospital emergency rooms have prepared cards with written questions to have ready for these situations.

Other Difficult Situations
In addition to not hearing your name called while waiting for tests or examinations, misunderstanding important

details of your diagnosis and prognosis, incorrectly interpreting specific questions concerning health care and medications, and missing what is being said when medical personnel are wearing surgical masks, you may find the following medical situations difficult and should be prepared to address them:

- When you are having a procedure related to your eyes, you may need special consideration because people with hearing loss need to see in order to understand what is being said.
- When your back is to the speaker, such as when you are in bed, receiving an injection, or being pushed in a wheelchair or on a gurney, you will need to remind personnel that you need to see them in order to understand them.
- When having a chest X-ray, ask the radiology technician to flash a light to let you know when to hold your breath.

Items to Ask for During a Hospital Stay

Hospitals are required by the Americans with Disabilities Act and Section 504 of the Rehabilitation Act to have assistive listening devices, such as one-on-one communicators, on the premises for their use. You may wish to ask for a telephone with a visible alert, an amplified telephone, or a TTY; a caption decoder for TV; and an International Symbol of Access for Hearing Loss for the door of your room.

Items to Take to the Hospital with You

Several items can be helpful in making your hospital stay less stressful:

- A small night light to facilitate speechreading at night
- A supply of SHHH Communication Tips to distribute to hospital personnel
- Your personal communication equipment

- Extra hearing aid batteries
- A storage container labeled with your name for your hearing aids
- A pen and paper to use when you are not able to wear your hearing aids

33

HEARING
WHEN TRAVELING

Travel is an enjoyable option, particularly during retirement years. As a hard of hearing person, traveling alone or with others does not need to be stressful. The secret to successful travel is anticipation and assertiveness. Think about what you need in order to feel safe and to remain independent when away from home. Before you leave home, plan strategies for getting what you need.

Away from home, you will have many opportunities to interact for the first time with strangers, including service providers, vendors, and other travelers. If you let them know at the outset that you do not hear well and what they can do to make communication easier, you will find that most people are happy to work with you to facilitate understanding.

Hotels and Motels
When making your reservation. In addition to inquiring about such things as king-size beds and the cost of an extra cot, request specific accommodations such as amplified telephones and TTYs, alerting devices, and closed-captioned TV. A number of equipment distributors work with hoteliers and hospitality franchises nationwide to make their establishments hearing accessible. Some of the equipment is permanently installed in rooms; other items are quickly installed after check-in. If the facility does not have these items, remind the manager that the Americans with Disabilities Act requires hotels and motels with five or more sleeping rooms to provide reasonable accommodations, including those mentioned above.

On arrival. If you have not requested these beforehand, request amplified telephones, alerting devices, and closed-captioned TV. If the establishment has this equipment, ask to have it installed in your room. It doesn't hurt to commend the establishment for providing these items.

Check-in also provides an opportunity to educate staff about ways to communicate with hard of hearing people. Because the registration area is usually noisy, ask personnel to face you and speak clearly (see Key 24).

Using the telephone. The telephone is essential for most travelers. Hotels are required to carry accessible telephones, but this could be a telephone in the lobby. Inquire about telephones when you make your reservations. If the establishment does not have accessible telephones in the room, consider going elsewhere. If, however, you must stay at a particular establishment and the hotel cannot provide a hearing aid-compatible telephone or an amplified handset, you may wish to carry a portable telephone amplifier with you. Some travelers like to carry a portable TTY (see Key 19).

Watching television. In the United States, hotels with five or more sleeping rooms are supposed to have captioned television in four percent of the rooms. If you need a decoder, request that one be hooked up in your room.

On Tour (Guided and On Your Own)

Traveling in groups does not have to be a frustrating experience for the hard of hearing person. When on a guided tour, position yourself as close as possible to the guide in order to maximize what you hear and also to see the guide's lip movements. If you own a portable FM system, bring it with you and ask the guide to use it. Explain how it works and show the guide how to wear the microphone. Some Scandinavian countries frequently have induction loops on tour buses. In art galleries and museums and at historic places, ask if you may borrow the guidebook used by guides, if available, or if you might use the written script for the audiotapes for self-guided tours.

Making Travel More Accessible in the Future

Accessibility in public places improves daily because people with disabilities, including hard of hearing people, are requesting access. If you need support services, ask for them. You also should praise people in places that do provide services. When you see a need for improvement, offer constructive criticism and recommendations. You can make a difference by offering suggestions such as: "If the video were captioned, it could be better understood by people with hearing loss and those who speak a language other than English." Because many national parks are working to upgrade facilities for people with hearing loss, inquire about the status, and use the equipment so that they will continue to work to accommodate hard of hearing people.

Traveling in a Car

Whether you are the driver or the passenger, you likely will want to converse with companions on long trips while keeping your eyes on the road. A one-on-one communicator will enable you to carry on a conversation easily (see Key 17). If you have an audio jack on your car radio, a neck loop enables you to listen to the radio or taped book.

Safety is always important. If you are not able to hear sirens or your signal light when driving, you could be placing yourself in a dangerous situation unnecessarily. Two signaling devices can help you. An emergency response indicator is a signaling device for the automobile that turns on a light when emergency vehicles such as fire, police, or ambulance sirens or car horns are nearby. A turn signal reminder can alert you that your left-right signal is "on." Several automobile manufacturers offer a rebate for the complete cost of these devices to hard of hearing and deaf people who have purchased a car manufactured after 1994.

Traveling on an Airplane

It is not easy for a hard of hearing person to hear in noisy places, and airports and airplanes can be especially noisy. When all goes well, the signs in the airport provide sufficient information about flight times, gate numbers, cancellations, and locations. However, the unexpected, such as a gate change or a delay, usually announced on a loudspeaker, can cause problems for the hard of hearing person. Gate personnel don't always remember that you have told them that you do not hear well and to alert you to important messages. One way to keep informed is to ask a fellow traveler on the same flight to inform you of such announcements. On the plane, you can give the flight attendant a written note with your name and seat number on it.

On the airplane, hearing the safety and evacuation procedures, the menu options, and announcements by the pilot can be difficult. Again, a written note to the flight attendant with your name and seat number is one way to solve this problem. You also can ask your seatmate to alert you if any unexpected announcements are made. If you do not hear well, you are not supposed to sit in the exit rows where you would be responsible for evacuation procedures in case of emergency. Commuter flights pose an additional problem because several flights leave from one gate and you must constantly be on the alert for changes. Whether you can or cannot hear announcements, remember to turn off FM equipment during take-off and landing because it interferes with the radio transmission between tower and cockpit.

People with hearing loss often experience a feeling of fullness or blockage when flying. This blockage of the ear, *barotitis*, which is caused by changes in atmospheric pressure, is both mild and reversible. The best thing you can do to avoid it is to not fly when you have a cold, or are undergoing an upper respiratory allergic reaction. If you must fly under either of the above conditions, or you know that your ears get blocked when flying, take a decongestant nasal spray with you and spray your nose two or three times one or two hours before landing.

If your ears start to feel blocked during landing, swallow repeatedly, sip some fluid, or hold your nose and try to "pop" your ears by blowing out gently while your mouth and nose are closed. If you have significant pain or hearing loss after landing, see your ear doctor.

Note: People with disabilities, including those with hearing loss, are eligible for the Golden Access Passport from the National Parks Service, which provides free entrance to recreational areas and parks in the United States.

Bon Voyage!

34

HEARING
IN THE COURTROOM

What would you do if you received a summons to report for jury duty?

You might take the easy way out and use your hearing loss as an excuse for not serving: If you can't hear the proceedings or the discussion among jurors, you would be violating the rights of the litigants; therefore, you can't serve. On the other hand, you might see jury service as a duty and a right to participate in our legal system. When you can't serve, you are denied equal access to our justice system.

If you are an advocate for the rights of hard of hearing people, you also may view jury duty as an opportunity to ensure that the courts are in compliance with the ADA (see Key 28). Most courthouses have installed ramps for people who need them and hired sign language interpreters for people who are deaf, but often they have no assistive listening devices to accommodate people who are hard of hearing.

Many court systems employ voice mail as the means for responding to the summons. This often is a difficult option for people with hearing loss. Although you can get a family member or friend to help you understand the message if you do not hear well on the telephone, or use the relay service, consider suggesting another method of responding to the commissioner of jurors, such as a return postcard.

Your response to the request to serve should include a statement such as: "I can serve if the facility has assistive listening systems, real-time captioning (see page 100), or devices in place to accommodate people who are hard of hearing." You also will need to state your specific needs.

At the courthouse, you may see signs posted outside a courtroom that indicate assistive listening devices are available. This does not mean that they are in every room of the courthouse or that they are in working condition. Very often, only one person in the court system is familiar with the devices—where they are kept, how they function, how to maintain them—and may not be available the day you are on jury duty. You may have to use your assertive skills to ensure that the system works for you before the proceedings begin. You must let them know what you need with ample notice.

The National Court Reporters Association launched a program, called Total Access Courtroom (TAC), to help make the courts become more accessible. Using the skills of court reporters, real-time captioning has become an accepted and desired tool in the courtroom. With this technology, the message can be displayed on a video monitor, printed out as a rough transcript, captured on a floppy disk, or printed in Braille seconds after information is transmitted by the court reporter to the computer.

At the same time you are ensuring that the courtroom is accessible, it is equally important that the jury deliberation room and other hearing rooms also are accessible. For a fair and impartial trial, you need to be privy to all communication.

Serving in other capacities. If you are a litigant or a witness in a trial, it is equally important for you to hear the proceedings. This is not the time to deny or hide your hearing loss; it is the time to speak up for what you need to serve the system well.

Officers of the Court
Attorneys, clerks, and judges also may experience hearing loss. In order to serve the judicial system, it is impor-

tant to hear the proceedings. As a responsible officer of the court, you know that this is not the time to hide a hearing loss. This is the time to take a leadership role by ensuring that the courtroom is accessible to you and to other people with hearing loss. Explore the options available to ensure a fair trial.

Other Legal Situations
It is essential that you understand what is being communicated during all aspects of the judicial system, including appearances in small claims court, observing a trial, and during everyday legal procedures such as preparing a will, settling an estate, and conducting real estate transactions, civil disputes, and tax preparation. Be sure to explain to your lawyer and others involved that you have a hearing loss and how they can best communicate with you.

This last advice applies outside the lawyer's office as well. It includes being upfront about your hearing loss in discussions with the social security office and other government agency personnel, or when being questioned by police officers and public officials.

35

VOLUNTEERING OR RETURNING TO WORK

Many people who retire from the work force often decide to return to work part-time or to engage in volunteer work. Your hearing loss should not deter you from either.

In the past, popular misconceptions about hearing loss were pervasive and strongly influenced decisions about whether firms and volunteer organizations recruited and hired hard of hearing people. Today, however, public attention to the nature and consequences of hearing loss never has been at a higher level.

The Americans with Disabilities Act specifies that employers cannot discriminate against qualified individuals with disabilities who, with reasonable accommodations, can perform essential functions of the position. Reasonable accommodations for hard of hearing people—such as accessible telephones, assistive devices in meeting rooms, job restructuring, and safety alerts—are relatively inexpensive and can enable you to do a job.

Remember that your previous training, background, and skills are more important than your hearing loss. Focus on what you can do, not on what might cause problems.

A number of practical strategies can help you overcome anxiety and get the work or volunteer position you want. The key to coping with hearing loss in the workplace is to be open about your hearing loss and let others know how best to communicate with you so you may achieve your highest potential and contribute your talent.

Employers and volunteer organizations may have little experience working with people with hearing loss. Even though you may be nervous, being open and honest about your hearing loss may help to enhance others' comfort level and ensure a smooth interview.

The interview presents an opportunity to show that although you have a hearing loss, you can still function well and do the job. This is no time to hide your hearing loss. If you need assistive devices and own them, take them with you. If you need assistive devices that you do not own but are necessary for you to function effectively on the job, you should request them up front so that your communication needs with employer or volunteer agency are clear from the beginning.

Once you are hired or accepted for a volunteer position, demonstrate your commitment by the quality and quantity of the work you perform and your work ethic.

In order to ensure that you have understood what you are supposed to do on the job, confirm instructions after they are given. You might ask for instructions in writing if this is more comfortable for you.

Often, meetings, training sessions, and small conferences are situations in which it is difficult to hear. Do something about this early on. Unresolved communication difficulties, whether with co-workers, other volunteers, supervisors, or clients, can make you look inefficient and incapable of carrying out your responsibilities.

Vocational Rehabilitation

You may wish to investigate your eligibility for vocational rehabilitation (VR) services. VR is the nationwide federal/state program that helps people with disabilities obtain appropriate training so that they can secure employment. All states, territories, and trust areas have a vocational rehabilitation agency. To be eligible for VR services, you must, among other requirements, have a physical or mental impairment that is a substantial impediment to employment.

36

A NEW FRIEND: THE INTERNET

Hearing aids, assistive devices, coping strategies, and healthy living are at the top of the list for people with hearing loss. There is, however, another device you may not have considered, but one that can help you communicate easily and bring the world to your doorstep: a personal computer (PC) with a program that gives you access to the Internet and electronic mail. Computers can be the answer to many of the communication difficulties you encounter daily as a person who is hard of hearing.

If you already have embraced computers, you are on the way to having another means of communicating easily with family members, friends, banks, airlines, and businesses, to name a few. The world is at your fingertips.

You may be hesitant, however. "Computers are expensive," you might say. They are—but well worth the investment when you realize all that you can do to facilitate communication. The new Net PCs cost less, and a used rebuilt computer is another alternative.

But, you may argue, "I don't even know how to type." You are never too old to learn, and hunting and pecking, although slower than ten-finger typing—the new word is keyboarding, by the way—enables you to become computer literate while picking up speed.

Ways to Use Your Computer
You may ask, "What can I do with a computer that I can't do with my old typewriter?" You can write personal and business letters or prepare newsletters and organize pre-

sentations for your volunteer work, all the tasks for which you use a typewriter, but you can do these with less frustration and you can do so many other things.

- A most valuable use of the computer for older Americans is keeping in touch with family and friends. When the telephone becomes a barrier to good communication because you are asking the person on the other end of the line to repeat, or when you are having difficulty understanding the voices of grandchildren and you want to say the right thing in order to keep your relationship with them meaningful, a computer and an electronic mail (e-mail) program could be the answer.

- Although hearing the voices of family members and being able to discern their moods from the tone is certainly a preferred way to communicate, e-mail provides a new world for people with hearing loss. It also keeps you from playing telephone tag. When you can leave a message with someone who has the information you need and receive an answer in writing, why spend time calling and struggling to hear the answer?

- If you use a TTY and would like to communicate with friends who have computers or if you use a computer and would like to communicate with friends who use a TTY, you might consider a computer with special equipment that allows it to function as a TTY. This feature may add to the cost, but if staying in touch is a priority for you, spend the money.

- You may be able to equip your computer with a special modem—a device that allows your computer to use telephone lines to transmit information to other computers or terminals equipped with compatible modems—to make it function as a TTY.

- The Internet also will provide you with an opportunity to participate in discussion groups and chat rooms, a new way of gaining and sharing information, making new friends with similar interests, and socializing.

- You can track your finances, and even do your banking and check writing. You can get the latest stock market information, track your investments, and buy and sell.
- If you enjoy games, a wealth of software is available in this area. If you are interested in genealogy, programs exist that make the organizing of information easy.
- If travel is high on your priority list, the Internet provides extensive information about places to visit, what there is to see, hotels and motels, and how best to get there. Airline scheduling, booking tickets, finding reduced rates—all are at your fingertips.
- If you have arthritis in addition to your hearing loss, and find that writing is painful, a computer keyboard may relieve the stress of corresponding with loved ones or for business purposes.
- And if you are interested in returning to work, or finding a part-time position, computer skills combined with your other skills and experience, could put you back in the workplace with a new career.

A word of warning. The technology in the field of computers is burgeoning and changes daily. The day you buy a computer, it will be out of date. But don't let that keep you from considering one—it can keep you connected, informed, and in touch with the world.

If you already own a computer and can access the World Wide Web, find out the latest information about hearing loss by visiting <http://www.shhh.org>.

37

HEARING LOSS AND ELDERCARE

With people living longer, many of them with multiple disabilities, the need for eldercare is expected to increase. Because fewer potential family members will be available to serve as caregivers for those needing long-term care, the demand for the services provided by nursing homes and adult day care centers is expected to escalate.

If someone you know has a hearing loss and is living in a nursing home, your role as a friend or relative is essential. You can provide a valuable service by becoming an advocate. Nursing home residents have rights and responsibilities, and unless they are in a nonresponsive state, they should be informed about their medical treatment and decisions related to their health problems. When residents don't understand what is happening, their apprehension rises to abnormal proportions.

People who lose their hearing late in life concomitant with the aging process are extremely sensitive and vulnerable to the denial syndrome for they view hearing loss as tangible evidence of aging or decline.

For some older people, who are living in nursing homes, hearing loss may have contributed to their placement in a long-term care facility. Communication problems such as inappropriate answers or apparent lack of response may be mistaken for mental confusion or loss of mental acuity.

Communication by staff members with residents who have hearing loss takes time and effort and often has a low priority. Since nursing homes are short staffed, residents with hearing loss often experience subtle, imagined, and even blatant discrimination for a variety of reasons ranging from lack of understanding on the part of staff members, misdiagnosis, or sheer lack of staff time for special efforts to communicate effectively, to impatience with the resident's refusal to admit a hearing problem.

Individuals who approach old age with negative feelings and at the same time have to deal with a progressive hearing loss are ill-equipped with coping skills for handling the accompanying prejudice/discrimination or for understanding the thoughtless stigmatization even among their peers.

Nursing homes would do well to become knowledgeable about the psychosocial effects of hearing loss on the individual (see Key 38). By recognizing that an isolating hearing loss—alone or in combination with other health problems such as diminished vision, manual dexterity, and memory loss—can increase a resident's anxiety, dependency, frustration, confusion, suspicion, and depression.

Providing Information
The following simple but relevant pieces of information you provide to nursing home staff members can greatly improve the comfort, adjustment, and mental health of the resident with hearing loss.
1. Ensure that the staff members know that the resident is hard of hearing. Educate them. Tell them how to communicate by giving them specific strategies such as "try to get the resident's attention before speaking." It is often helpful to flick the light switch on and off to alert the resident that someone is entering the room. You may need to repeat this information because staff members may forget, and you may be communicating with different personnel on different shifts. Be patient and polite, but be persistent.
2. Alert staff members to the fact that the resident does not understand messages over the intercom. Ask that

information specific for the resident be delivered face to face. You might suggest that a note or the access symbol be posted at the nurses' station as a reminder when communicating important general information. Remind staff members that even though people with hearing loss use their eyes to make up for what they cannot hear, most people who lose their hearing later in life are not skilled speechreaders, and only 30 to 40 percent of speech is visible on the lips.

3. Residents who have difficulty understanding conversation or instructions, ask for frequent repetition, turn the radio or television on too loud, can't understand on the telephone, and cup a hand to the ear may be experiencing additional hearing loss. You can remind the staff to check for a buildup of earwax and have it removed. If hearing does not improve, you can suggest that a hearing evaluation may be in order. Many nursing homes have a consulting audiologist who is available on call to evaluate hearing loss and hearing aids.

4. If the resident wears a hearing aid, you can ensure that it is in proper working order and that an adequate supply of batteries is on hand. You might instruct staff members that a daily check of the hearing aid should be as much a part of the morning and bedtime patient care as the cleaning of dentures and washing of eyeglasses. Staff members should know how to turn the aid on and off, set the volume control, and replace weak or dead batteries.

Many of the recommended procedures for a hospital stay discussed in Key 32 also apply to nursing home residency.

38

OVERCOMING PSYCHOSOCIAL EFFECTS OF HEARING LOSS

The loss, even partial, of the sense of hearing, upon which much of our interpersonal communication is based, can be described as a major life loss. It is much different from hearing loss that is present at birth or begins in early childhood, particularly from a psychosocial perspective, because it can cause changes in your job, marriage, and entire lifestyle. When you lose your hearing in adulthood, you experience a kind of deprivation, the loss of a sense you have always taken for granted. The multidimensional effects of that loss can alter the way you feel about yourself as well as the way you think others feel about you.

Your personality does not change because you lose your hearing. Someone who is naturally quiet and reserved may experience their hearing loss quite differently than someone who is friendly and outgoing by nature. Because you are unique, you will experience hearing loss in your own way, however, some predictable behaviors are common to people who experience the onset of hearing loss as adults. It helps to understand those behaviors because they validate many of the feelings you have about yourself and about how other people react and respond to you. Understanding can also motivate you to help yourself develop coping strategies that work.

Hearing loss may create a communication barrier between you and other people. Spontaneity in conversation may become difficult because your brain needs to work overtime to process information and fill in the missing pieces of the conversation puzzle. Your ability to cope with these changes will affect the way your hearing loss affects your life from a psychosocial perspective.

Perceptions

Your self-image and the image you convey to others are based heavily on perceptions, but sometimes perceptions do not reflect reality. For example, you may believe that only old people wear hearing aids, that hearing loss is a sign of old age. That belief alone may prevent you from admitting you have a hearing loss. Other people may have perceptions about you that portray you very differently from who you really are. If you do not respond to other people when or as expected, they will form perceptions that define the way they think about you. If you conceal your hearing loss, there is nothing to indicate those perceptions are wrong. People will define you by their faulty perceptions rather than by reality. They may even choose not to acknowledge you in the future because they believe you chose to be unfriendly to them in the past. This kind of seesaw can create hurt feelings for everyone. Hard of hearing people often feel that "nobody understands," them, which may be partially true but is all too often interpreted as "nobody likes me." This belief can lead to mild and even more serious levels of depression.

Denial

If you refuse to admit you cannot hear well and persist in blaming other people for not speaking clearly or loudly enough, you are in a psychological state known as denial. When you are in denial you cannot seek help for your hearing loss; in fact, you become quite helpless. When you choose this negative coping strategy, you will fool no one but yourself. If the people who know you don't guess that you have a hearing problem, they will wonder why you act or react strangely. People whom you meet for the first time may perceive you as aloof, dull, or even mentally inferior. Their conclusions about your unusual behavior have the potential to be far more damaging than the upfront knowledge that you simply don't hear well.

Avoidance

As time passes, you may find yourself avoiding situations in which hearing is difficult, as well as certain people whose voices you know you have difficulty understanding. Avoidance is a negative coping strategy that will gradually erode your ties to people and activities that you formerly enjoyed. Avoidance leads to different degrees of withdrawal from your former way of life—on the job, with friends and in leisure activities—and within your immediate family. In fact, you can effectively isolate yourself from the many joys of parenting and grandparenting if you choose to avoid having to listen to your younger family members who have higher-pitched (and more difficult to understand) voices, rather than getting help for your hearing.

The reasons for denial run the gamut from negative cultural attitudes to ignorance about the nature of hearing loss itself. You deny because you don't understand the physiology of hearing loss. Because you are confused, you cannot possibly tell other people how to help you. When denial becomes chronic and long lasting, your hearing problem will intensify because it becomes a problem for everyone. If you become angry and defiant when the subject of hearing loss is brought up, you will create a standoff that nobody can win. Others become frustrated and may even go so far as to begin avoiding you.

Self-imposed isolation that eventually results from denial can lead to loneliness. But it is not necessary to live a lonely life if you admit you have a hearing loss and do whatever you need to do to help yourself hear better. If your associates believe you could help yourself but choose not to, they may lose patience with you. On the other hand, you will find that most people will go out of their way to learn effective communication strategies if they know you are helping yourself as best you can.

Self help. Self help combines accepting your hearing loss and using appropriate technology along with a willingness to become educated about the causes of and potential strategies for living with hearing loss. Self help may mean being fitted with a hearing aid and learning the basics of speechreading. It could mean that you use assistive devices that go beyond your hearing aid. It may mean learning cued speech or some other form of manual communication. The myriad options available to you can make a positive difference when you open your mind to learning about them and adapting them to your needs.

Other Negative Behaviors
You learned the difference between aggressive, assertive, and passive communication in Key 23.

Aggressiveness is a common reaction to the frustrations caused by hearing loss, but an aggressive person makes demands that cross boundaries and interfere with the rights of other people. For example, if you insist on having the television at your preferred loudness level rather than using one of the many assistive devices that enable you to control the volume without creating an environment that is too loud for everyone else, you are exhibiting aggressive controlling behavior.

Monopolizing is another example of aggressive behavior. This behavior is more common among people who have always been gregarious and outgoing. The monopolizer controls conversations by dominating them. The logic is simple: If you do all the talking, you won't have to listen; therefore, you will know what is being discussed. Needless to say, this behavior will become tiresome for others and your associates may cope with this behavior by avoiding you.

Passive behavior can be as devastating as aggressive behavior. Passive people do not complain nor do they seek help; they simply accept the hearing loss as a fact of life. The psychosocial implications of passive behavior vary depending on the innate personality of the individual.

Assertiveness is the middle ground between aggressiveness and passivity. When you are assertive, you learn how to help yourself as well as to help other people help you. You may learn to find some humor in the mistakes you make. You also accept the reality that you will, on occasion, experience feelings of being "left out" of conversations and decision making. These times will still be hurtful, but you learn not to let your feelings interfere with your personal interactions with others. How you assert yourself when this happens will have a direct bearing on the cooperation you receive from others.

Fear

Considerable fear may be attached to hearing loss. Fear may arise because you become concerned about how your hearing loss is going to affect your way of life. If you are employed, the fear of losing your job may be extremely stressful. Hard of hearing people are constantly faced with the fear of misunderstanding and misinterpreting incoming information. Fear can lead to chronic worry and anxiety.

Fear is the emotion that is biologically designed to elicit the human body's stress response. The stress response, often called the "fight or flight response," is biologically designed to help you fight off or run away from the impending danger of a life-threatening situation. Rarely does hearing loss create a life-threatening situation, yet many hard of hearing people live in an unhealthy state of chronic stress because they feel constantly threatened. Learning effective methods of managing stress should be one of your personal goals (see Key 39).

39

HEALTHY LIVING/ MANAGING STRESS

All people experience good and bad stress. At its best, stress serves to invigorate, motivate, and give you the personal power and strength to achieve and excel. At its worst, stress will cause the systems within your body to chronically overwork. Stress becomes a concern when it is chronic and poorly managed.

By now you know that hearing loss can be stressful. You also know that your physical and emotional well-being depends on how you learn to manage the hearing loss and stress in your life. When your body's stress response is triggered, several physical reactions take place, including increased cardiac output, breathing, and blood pressure. You may feel your heart pound and experience shortness of breath. Under stress, your muscles will tense because blood flows to them to provide you with extra physical strength. These bodily responses are obvious to you. All of these normal responses are intended to help you face situations that are potentially life threatening. This is why the stress response is often called the "fight or flight response."

Your bodily responses to negative stress create symptoms. When your muscles tense up you may experience pain, most often in the shoulders, neck, and legs. Most headache pain is the result of muscle tension. Your digestive tract may react with constipation, diarrhea, or pain from spasms. Because your breathing rate increases you may perspire and experience dry mouth. The stress response creates different symptoms in different people.

Take a moment to think about what happens to your body and mind when you feel stressed or fearful. You will recognize the effects as you personally experience them.

Stressors

The stress response kicks in when a demand, situation (real or perceived), or circumstance disrupts your normal state of equilibrium. Whatever elicits the stress response is called a *stressor*. Stressors may be perceived rather than real. Worry is a huge stressor for most people. If you spend time worrying about situations that may or may not occur because you are afraid of how you will cope with your hearing loss if they happen, you are dealing with a perceived stressor. It's much like worrying for days ahead about a trip to the dentist. The real event is far less traumatic than the perceived and imagined event that caused you to worry and feel stressed for days. It is not healthy to expend time and energy with the stressor called "worry." In fact, it can actually do harm if you don't learn to control it.

Stress Management

A successful stress management program will require a two-pronged approach that includes both stress prevention and stress management. You will want to adopt a holistic approach that incorporates time management, good nutrition, a drug-free lifestyle, exercise, and relaxation strategies all of which are vital components of an effective stress management program. When you minimize the amount of stress in your life, and the effects of stress on your body, you will discover that you can also manage your hearing loss well.

Time management. Time management is a key to stress management. Schedule time for work and play by balancing the daily routine. Recreational activities that you enjoy can serve as a great source of stress release. Don't overprogram yourself, but don't use your hearing loss as an excuse to say no when you really should say yes. Rest and relaxation should be important parts of your schedule. If you enjoy volunteer work be sure to include it in your schedule.

Good nutrition. Diet and lifestyle have an indirect effect on hearing loss. Both hearing loss and tinnitus typically become temporarily worse when one is fatigued, under stress, and malnourished. Although these changes are transient, their effects may influence your general sense of well-being. As with any medical problem, the better your diet, the more adequate your rest, and the better your sense of well-being, the less effect the hearing loss will have on you.

- *Low salt.* When you reduce fluid retention in your body you also reduce the fluid in your inner ear. The buildup of fluid, associated with tinnitus and Ménière's, can be reduced with appropriate control of salt in your diet.
- *Low fat.* If you have hyperlipidemia (excessive amounts of fat and fatty substances in the blood), you also may have inner ear symptoms such as tinnitus, dizziness, and fullness in the ears. By following a dietary regime to reduce or eliminate the cardiovascular risk factors, the inner ear symptoms may also diminish or disappear.
- *No caffeine.* For many people caffeine can be a stimulant. If you are experiencing stress, you may want to cut back on your intake. Remember, caffeine is present not only in coffee and tea, but in soft drinks and chocolate as well.

Medications. Drugs often are prescribed to relieve stress, but they do not relieve the underlying cause; they can even create more stress. If you take several medications—over the counter and those prescribed for you—try to get all your medications through one doctor, your internist preferably. Many medications are ototoxic and combinations can cause other problems (see Key 8).

Exercise. Whether you engage in an activity as easy as walking or something more strenuous, physical exercise can relieve tension and relax you. Exercise also increases blood flow to the ears, which is known to improve hearing. Breathing, a relaxation technique described below, is often considered the number one exercise.

Relaxation

When your body is chronically stressed, it experiences continuous wear and tear with little or no rest. It doesn't take a great deal of physiological knowledge to understand why it is not healthy to allow your body to remain in a stressed state for long periods of time. Therefore, it is very important for you to learn how to allow your body to return to its normal level of functioning which is called *homeostasis*. To do this, you must learn to elicit your body's natural stress fighting mechanism, the relaxation response.

Relaxation is the exact opposite of stress. Your body cannot be relaxed and stressed at the same time. Relaxation, which begins with proper breathing, is the key to managing stress. For most people today, true relaxation is a learned skill rather than a natural one.

You may remember learning about diaphragmatic breathing when you were a child in grade school. You probably even practiced it then. Most likely you have forgotten all about the rudiments of proper breathing; now you either do it naturally or you do not. In fact, you may not even be able to describe the way you breathe even when you think about it. Proper breathing can be visualized. Picture your lungs as a glass and your breath as water. When water is poured into a glass it fills from the bottom up. When water goes out of the glass it empties from the top down. That is exactly how proper breathing works. Experiment by visualizing it that way.

The breathing cycle has three phases: inhalation, pause, and exhalation. The inhalation phase is the tension-producing phase. As you awaken from sleep or a relaxed state, it is normal to yawn, stretch, and take a deep breath simultaneously. The muscular tension created produces a feeling of invigoration, refreshment, mental stimulation, and alertness. When you practice relaxation techniques, you will use the inhalation phase to bring yourself out of a relaxed state.

The exhalation phase of the breathing cycle is the relaxation phase. During exhalation you let go of the tension that developed naturally in the body from inhalation. The exhalation phase is the built-in mechanism for relaxation that everyone has. Exhalation normally is felt as a downward movement because the muscles relax and gravity causes you to sink down. The sensations identified with exhalation—feelings of heaviness, slowing down, letting go, comfort, and contentment—are exactly opposite of the sensations of inhalation. These sensations can be easily identified and sensed. When practicing relaxation techniques, you will concentrate on the exhalation phase and disregard the inhalation phase. Begin your relaxation program now by concentrating on your breathing rhythm. Practice this for a few minutes several times during the day. You should not fall asleep during this exercise. Remember to bring yourself out of the relaxed state by inhaling deeply and stretching. When you are breathing properly, you will feel refreshed after only a few minutes of practicing this exercise. Try it the next time you are faced with a stressor.

Once you have mastered the release of tension through proper breathing you will want to learn about other stress management techniques such as progressive relaxation, total body relaxation, and imaging. Your local library has many books that will provide you with step-by-step instructions on how to master these techniques. You may even find a class through a local health center that offers instruction in relaxation. One word of caution for people with hearing loss: Relaxation works best when you are comfortable closing your eyes. If you need to speechread a group leader, you may find the group setting uncomfortable, even stressful. Be sure the group leader understands your needs. Better yet, find a relaxation program especially designed for hard of hearing people. Self Help for Hard of Hearing People, Inc., often includes such a session in the annual convention programming. Participants then take the information home to share with other hard of hearing people.

40

WHAT IS SHHH?

Self Help for Hard of Hearing People, Inc. (SHHH) is a nonprofit educational organization dedicated to the well-being of people of all ages and communication styles who do not hear well. The largest international consumer organization of its kind, SHHH and its members are catalysts who make mainstream society more accessible to people who are hard of hearing. They accomplish this through education, advocacy, and self help.

The SHHH national office in Bethesda, Maryland, provides information and education on many aspects of hearing loss—from technological and medical advances to coping and parenting strategies—through publications, resource materials, and an annual convention that offers workshops and opportunities to try out new technology.

SHHH's award-winning bimonthly magazine, *Hearing Loss: The Journal of Self Help for Hard of Hearing People*, has a readership of 200,000 and is the only educational journal for hard of hearing people in America. The unwritten theme of "Hearing Loss: You Can Do Something About It" permeates the pages of each issue. Authors are people of various backgrounds—renowned professionals in the hearing health industry, psychologists, doctors, scientists, and educators. Other popular articles are personal narratives written by SHHH members.

SHHH's knowledgeable staff members represent the interests of people with hearing loss, and advocate for full access to services for them in government, professional, academic, private sector, and research forums. SHHH supports medical research, new technology, and legislation that will alleviate the effects of hearing loss. Together with its members, the organization worked toward the passage of the Americans with Disabilities Act, developed guidelines relating to hearing access, and continues to encourage provision of appropriate accommodations at the local level.

SHHH and its members believe that people with hearing loss can help themselves and one another to participate fully and successfully in society. They recognize that in order to remain in control of their lives, people with hearing loss must first educate themselves, and then their families, friends, co-workers, teachers, hearing health care providers, people in industry and government, and others with whom they interact. SHHH philosophy emphasizes that informed consumers make better decisions about the options available to them and are able to address hearing loss more effectively than people who do not have such information available.

SHHH has 250 chapters nationwide whose members meet regularly to learn about hearing loss from one another as well as from professionals in the field (see Appendix A). Like the national organization, local chapters emphasize that with education, information, shared experience, and support, people with hearing loss can develop strategies for living successfully. Chapter members also advocate for access in the workplace, hotels, schools, court systems, and medical and entertainment facilities in order to help make their communities and states more accessible for people with hearing loss.

For more information, contact:
Self Help for Hard of Hearing People, Inc.
7910 Woodmont Avenue, Suite 1200
Bethesda, MD 20814
(301) 657-2248 (Voice)
(301) 657-2249 (TTY)
FAX: (301) 913-9413
URL: http://www.shhh.org

41

SOME FINAL WORDS

Over the nearly 25 years that I have lived with hearing loss, I have learned a few lessons:

- Hearing loss can cause frustration but with education and proper attitude, the frustration and the disability can be lessened.
- Responsive and experienced hearing health care providers are worth their weight in gold.
- Support groups are essential.
- Family members, friends, and co-workers can provide a large measure of support, but they need to be educated to your needs and you to theirs.
- The market is full of assistive devices that should be explored and used.
- The technology used in hearing aids and assistive devices is burgeoning and improving.

The Importance of Communication

We all need to communicate effectively. In order to do this, I have a few suggestions:

- Learn as much as possible about your own hearing loss.
- Learn what services are best provided by otolaryngologists, audiologists, and hearing aid specialists, and choose the professional who best provides the service you need.
- Together with your hearing health care specialist, evaluate hearing aids and get the one—two if recommended—that best meets your needs.
- Learn assertive techniques to use with family members and other people, such as "It would help me to understand you, if you faced me when you spoke" and "I can

be a part of this conversation if only one of you speaks at a time."

- Find other sources of support, as well. It is important to meet other people with similar hearing losses, and these people may be found through membership in groups such as SHHH.
- Learn some basic sign language; if nothing else, learn the alphabet. On my first trip abroad after I lost my hearing, I taught my daughter to fingerspell the alphabet. She then could help me with foreign names when I was having difficulty understanding them.
- Find out which assistive listening and alerting devices can help you in various situations. Keep abreast of the latest technology, since it changes rapidly.
- Keep your expectations for improvement realistic.
- And more important than everything else, keep your sense of humor.

GLOSSARY

ABC (Auditory Brainstem Response Audiometry) A hearing test in which a person's ability to hear "clicks" is determined by comparing a resting brain wave pattern with a brain waving pattern when "clicks" are made.

ADA (Americans with Disabilities Act) Public Law 101-336 passed in 1990 that prohibits discrimination on the basis of disability in employment, transportation, public accommodation, state and local government, and telecommunications.

Adventitiously deaf People who were born hearing and who lost their hearing later in life.

Alerting device Visual or tactile devices that alert a person who cannot hear to sounds such as door knocks, telephone rings, and fire alarms.

American Sign Language (ASL) See Sign language.

Amplified telephone A telephone that is equipped with volume control either built into the handset, the body of the telephone, or via an attachment.

Assistive listening device (ALD) A device that, used with or without a hearing aid, brings a speaker's voice directly to the ear of the person with hearing loss.

Assistive listening system (ALS) A system used in rooms of assembly and with large groups to make dialogue accessible (see Audio induction loop, Infrared, and FM).

Audiogram A graph on which a person's ability to hear different pitches of sound is recorded.

Audiologist A specialist in testing and evaluating hearing and providing nonmedical management of hearing loss, including hearing aids, assistive devices, and rehabilitation.

Audio induction loop   A coil of electrical wire that creates a magnetic field that can transmit sound and thus permit individuals with hearing loss to hear the sound without background noise or echoes.

Audiometer   A device for testing hearing.

Aural rehabilitation   Specialized training for people with hearing loss that includes speechreading, how to listen, how to speak.

Binaural   Refers to hearing with both ears.

Body aid   A powerful hearing aid used by people with profound hearing losses that consists of a transmitter, receiver, earmold, cord, and batteries.

BTE (behind-the-ear)   A hearing aid worn behind the ear that is connected to an earmold by thin plastic tubing.

Canal aid   See ITC (in-the-canal) aid.

Closed captions   Text of spoken dialogue and sounds displayed on TV and videos that is visible only to people using a caption decoder or TV with built-in decoder chip.

Cochlear implant   A surgically implanted electronic device that allows people with profound hearing loss to hear environmental sounds, improve speechreading, monitor their own speech, and often understand voices.

Conductive hearing loss   A hearing loss caused by damage to the outer or middle ear. This type of hearing loss often is correctable medically or surgically.

Congenitally deaf   Said of people who are born deaf or become deaf soon after birth.

CROS (Contralateral Routing of Signal)   A type of hearing aid often recommended when one ear has nearly normal hearing.

Cerumen   Earwax.

Cued speech   A sound-based visual communication system that uses eight handshapes in four different locations (cues) in combination with the natural mouth movements of speech.

DAI   See Direct audio input.

Deaf   A term that may be used to describe a person with severe or profound hearing loss.

Decibel (dB)   The unit used to measure the intensity or loudness of sound; the higher the dB, the louder the sound.

Decoder   An electronic device that reads a special code in the television signal and converts it to characters on the viewer's television screen.

Direct audio input   An option that bypasses the hearing aid's microphone by plugging a sound source directly into a hearing aid.

Earbud   A small transducer encased in a round foam rubber covering that is inserted into the ear canal. Like earphones, earbuds deliver sound to the ear, but many people think they are more comfortable than earphones.

Earmold   An acrylic or polyvinyl mold that couples the sound from the hearing aid to the ear.

E-Mail   Electronic mail, where messages are sent and received electronically; used by many computer owners.

Fingerspelling   Using handshapes to represent the letters of the alphabet.

Feedback   The squealing noise emitted when some of the amplified sound escapes from around an earmold or ITE and ITC hearing aids.

Frequency   The number of vibrations per second of a sound, usually expressed in Hz (hertz); the lower the Hz, the lower the pitch.

FM (Frequency Modulation) system   A device that transmits amplified sound by radio waves to a receiver, thus eliminating background noise and distance problems.

Hard of hearing   A term that may be used to describe a person with any degree of hearing loss, ranging from mild to profound, who can understand some speech sounds with or without a hearing aid.

Hearing aid   An electronic device used to amplify sound (see BTE, ITC, ITE).

Hearing Aid Compatibility Act of 1988   Act that mandates that all telephones manufactured in the United States from 1989 on should be hearing aid-compatible.

Hearing dog   A dog that has completed a training course to alert its owner to a variety of sounds in different environments.

Hearing health care provider   Audiologists, hearing aid specialists, and otolaryngologists.

Hearing loss   The loss of hearing ability, ranging from mild to profound.

Infrared system   A device that transmits amplified sound by invisible light waves to a receiver, thus eliminating background noise and distance problems.

International symbol of access for hearing loss   Symbol, used worldwide, that identifies locations where communication access is provided.

Interpreter   A person who conveys the spoken message to a person with hearing loss by the use of sign language (visible movements of hands, body, and face), orally (silently mouthing the words), or with cued speech.

ITC (in-the-canal) aid   The smallest of hearing aids consisting of an earmold and hearing aid as one unit, fitted to the ear canal.

ITE (in-the-ear) aid   A hearing aid consisting of an earmold and hearing aid as one unit, worn in the contour of the outer ear.

Lipreading   See Speechreading.

Mastoid   The rear portion of the temporal bone behind the ear.

Ménière's disease   A disease of the labyrinth of the ear, characterized by loss of hearing, ringing in the ears, and dizziness.

Monaural   Refers to hearing with one ear.

Neckloop   A loop of wire worn like a necklace that creates a magnetic field that can transmit sound when plugged into a portable radio or personal FM or infrared receiver.

Otolaryngologist A medical doctor who specializes in problems of the ear and throat.

Otologist A medical doctor who specializes in problems of the ear.

Presbycusis The slow, progressive type of hearing loss that often accompanies aging.

Real-time captioning The process of producing and projecting onto a screen verbatim dialogue as typed by a court reporter; clear, accurate print that is easily visible to people in large audiences.

Residual hearing The amount of hearing that remains after the occurrence of hearing loss.

Relay service Service that enables text telephone (TTY) users to communicate with non-text telephone users by way of a relay service communications assistant.

Sensorineural hearing loss Also called nerve deafness, a type of hearing loss caused by damage to the inner ear, auditory nerve, or auditory cortex of the brain; it is permanent and usually helped with hearing aids.

Sign language A manual system of communication by which spoken concepts and language are represented visually. Depending on personal preferences, deaf and hard of hearing people in the United States may choose to communicate using the unique grammar and syntax of American Sign Language (ASL) or another variety of signing that uses features taken from ASL and English.

Signed English A form of sign language that uses signs in English word order.

Silhouette An adapter, placed behind the ear and used with a hearing aid equipped with a T-switch, that transmits an FM radio signal to the aid.

Speechreading The interpretation of the spoken message by recognizing the movements of the lips, jaws, and tongue as well as additional cues such as body language, gestures, facial expressions, and conversational context.

Telecoil (T-switch)   A setting on a hearing aid used in conjunction with a hearing aid-compatible telephone, assistive listening device, and audio loop system that enables the hard of hearing person to hear better by eliminating disturbing background noise and the effect of distance.

Telecommunications relay service   See Relay service.

Text telephone   See TTY.

Tinnitus   Noise in the ears, such as ringing, clicking, buzzing, or roaring.

TTY (TDD and text telephone)   A telecommunication device that transmits and receives typewritten messages when used in conjunction with a telephone.

APPENDIX A

SHHH AFFILIATE LISTING

Self Help for Hard of Hearing People, Inc. has a nation-wide support network of affiliates that meet regularly to learn about hearing loss and coping strategies through self help. Local SHHH meetings offer:

- A place where your hearing loss is accepted and under-stood
- A communication-accessible stress-free environment
- An opportunity to share your concerns and learn from others
- Ways in which you can make a difference for yourself and others
- Support, referrals, and information
- Coping strategies and the latest technological informa-tion
- Enlightenment for family members, relatives, and friends
- Fellowship and friendship—listening ears and helping hands

If you would like to join an SHHH affiliate or start a new group, contact the SHHH national chapter develop-ment office. If you don't see an affiliate listed where you live, call SHHH and inquire (see Key 40).

Alabama
Birmingham*
Rocket City

Alaska
Fairbanks

Arizona
Greater Phoenix*
Sun City*

Arkansas
Little Rock*

California
Banning*
Barstow
Camarillo
Conejo Valley
Diablo Valley*
Escondido*
Fresno*
La Mesa
Livermore/Pleasanton/
　San Ramon*
Long Beach/Lakewood*
Los Angeles/Culver
　City*
Napa (North Bay)*
Oakland (East Bay)
Orange County*
Peninsula*
Redding/Anderson*

---

* Chapter
+ Seniors

Redlands
Sacramento*
San Diego (Sports Arena)
San Diego (Rancho
　Bernardo)
San Diego (Pacific Beach)
San Jose*
San Fernando Valley*
San Francisco*
Santa Barbara
Santa Maria Area*
Solano County
Ukiah
Ventura/Ojai

Colorado
Boulder*
Central Denver*

Connecticut
Central Connecticut*
East Haven

Delaware
Wilmington*

Florida
Boca Raton*
Bradenton
Clearwater/St. Petersburg*
Delray*
Fort Myers
Lauderdale Lakes*
Miami (Coral Gables)
Naples
North Port/Port Charlotte*

Okaloosa
Palm Beaches*
Pensacola
Port St. Lucie
Sarasota*
Sun City Center
Tampa

Georgia
Aiken-Augusta (Sc/GA)
Atlanta*
Gainesville-Lanier*
Rome

Hawaii
Honolulu*

Idaho
Boise*
Coeur d'Alene*
Moscow

Illinois
Chicago
  Loop*
  North Side*
  S. Suburban*
  W. Suburban*
Jacksonville
North Shore*+
Peoria*
Quad Cities (IL/IA)*
Springfield

Indiana
Evansville

Granger
South Bend
West Lafayette

Iowa
Des Moines*
Iowa City/Cedar Rapids
Quad Cities (IL/IA)*

Kansas
Johnson County
Kansas City (KS/MO)*

Kentucky
Kentucky Lake
Northern Kentucky
Louisville

Louisiana
Alexandria
New Orleans*
Northwest Louisiana*

Maryland
Annapolis
Bel Air*
Greater Baltimore*
Montgomery County*
Towson

Massachusetts
Attleboro
Cape Cod
Greater Boston*
Framingham
North of Boston

Plymouth/Duxbury
Springfield
South Shore
Worcester

Michigan
Birmingham
Gaastra
Grand Rapids
Jackson
Kalamazoo*
Lansing*
Muskegon*
Traverse City
Washtenaw Area*

Minnesota
Central Minnesota
 (St. Cloud)*
Minneapolis*
Southern Minnesota
 (Fairbault)

Mississippi
Biloxi
Jackson

Missouri
Kansas City (KS/MO)*
Lee's Summit
St. Joseph*
St. Louis*

Montana
Billings*
Bozeman

Nebraska
North Platte
Omaha*

Nevada
Las Vegas*

New Hampshire
Manchester/Concord/
 Nashua

New Jersey
Bergen County
Central Jersey*
Madison
Middlesex County
Northwest NJ
 (Long Valley)
South Jersey*

New Mexico
Albuquerque*
Roswell
Santa Fe

New York
Albany*
Corning*
Finger Lakes
Jamestown
Poughkeepsie*
Rochester
 (Day and Evening)*
Syracuse*
Utica*

Westchester*
Western NY (Buffalo)*
New York City Area
Brooklyn*
Huntington*
Manhattan*
North Shore (Roslyn)
South Nassau
  (Oceanside)*

North Carolina
Chapel Hill*
Charlotte*
Durham*
Greensboro
Hendersonville
Raleigh*
Wilmington
Winston-Salem*

Ohio
Canton Area*
Cincinnati*+
Cleveland Metro
Cleveland West
  (Rocky River)*
Columbus*
Lebanon+
Lima
Lorain County (Elyria)
Marion
Zanesville*

Oklahoma
Oklahoma City
  (Day/Evening)*

Oregon
Douglas County
Lane County (Eugene)*
Lowestin (Lake Oswego)
Medford
Portland*

Pennsylvania
Berks County
Delaware County
  (Springfield)*
Grove City
Harrisburg*
Lancaster*
Lebanon County
  (Cornwall)+
Lehigh Valley*
Montgomery County
Philadelphia #1*
Philadelphia (Center City)
Pittsburgh*
Schuylkill County
Squirrel Hill
Wyoming Valley
York Area

Rhode Island
Narragansett*
Providence*+

South Carolina
Aiken-Augusta (SC/GA)
Columbia*

South Dakota
Sioux Falls

Tennessee
Chattanooga*
Knoxville
  (East Tennessee)
Knoxville (Maryville)
Memphis

Texas
Amarillo
Austin
Corpus Christi
Dallas*
East Texas (Longview)
El Paso*
Fort Worth*
Houston*
San Antonio*

Utah
Salt Lake City Area

Vermont
Burlington
Montpelier
Rutland

Virginia
Fredericksburg*
Northern Virginia*
Roanoke
Sterling/Leesburg

Williamsburg*
Winchester

Washington
Edmonds
Everett
Everson
Horizon House
  (Seattle)+
Kitsap
Lacey
Lake Washington
Port Angeles
Sedro Wolley
Seattle Hear Here*
West Seattle*
South King County*
Tacoma*

Wisconsin
Stevens Point*
Fond du Lac*
Appleton*
Madison Area*
Milwaukee Metro*
Minocqua
Waukesha*
Whitewater

Wyoming
Casper

APPENDIX B

INFORMATION RESOURCES ON HEARING LOSS

In addition to Self Help for Hard of Hearing People, Inc. (SHHH), the organizations listed below provide information of interest to people with hearing loss.

Academy of Dispensing Audiologists (ADA)
3008 Millwood Avenue
Columbia, SC 29205

ADA represents audiologists who dispense hearing aids as part of their audiological and rehabilitative practice.

American Academy of Audiology (AAA)
8201 Greensboro Drive, # 300
McLean, VA 22102

AAA is a nonprofit organization for professional audiologists that serves as a forum for exchange of information and ideas in the areas of current research, clinical practices, hearing aid amplification/cochlear implants, and comprehensive rehabilitative intervention for people with hearing loss. AAA provides listings of certified audiologists to the general public.

**American Academy of Otolaryngology—
   Head and Neck Surgery, Inc. (AAO–HNS)**
One Prince Street
Alexandria, VA 22314

AAO–HNS is a nonprofit medical society that represents the majority of otolaryngologists in the United States. AAO–HNS provides patient education leaflets and physician listings to the public.

The American Association of Speech-Language Pathology and Audiology (ASHA)
10801 Rockville Pike
Rockville, MD 20852-3259

ASHA is the professional, scientific, and accrediting organization for speech-language pathologists and audiologists. ASHA provides information about communication disorders, as well as listings of certified speech-language pathologists and audiologists to the general public.

American Tinnitus Association (ATA)
P.O. Box 5
Portland, OR 97207

ATA provides information about tinnitus, and referrals to local hearing professional and support groups nationwide.

HEAR NOW
9745 E. Hampden Avenue
Suite 300
Denver, CO 80231-4923

HEAR NOW is a national, charitable organization that raises funds to provide hearing aids, cochlear implants, and related services to people with hearing loss who do not have the resources to purchase their own devices.

National Information Center on Deafness (NICD)
Gallaudet University
800 Florida Avenue, N.E.
Washington, D.C. 20002-3695

NICD is a centralized source of up-to-date objective information on topics dealing with deafness and hearing loss. The center collects, develops, and disseminates information about all aspects of hearing loss and services offered to deaf and hard of hearing people nationwide.

National Institute on Deafness and Other
Communication Disorders Heredity Hearing
Impairment Resource Registry (NIDCD-HHIRR)
555 N. 30th Street
Omaha, NE 68131

HHIRR, a national resource in the study of hereditary hearing loss including advances about research, collects information from individuals with hearing loss, and matches families with appropriate research projects.

National Institute on Deafness and Other
Communication Disorders (NIDCD) Clearinghouse
P.O. Box 3777
Washington, D.C. 20013-7777

NIDCD Clearinghouse is an information service for health professionals, patients, people in industry and business, and consumers, about the areas of hearing, balance, smell, taste, voice, speech, and language. The clearinghouse focuses on the medical and pathological aspects of deafness and other communication disorders, and offers a database of references to journal articles, books, audiovisual materials, brochures, and other educational materials. It also offers information packets, directories, and a newsletter.

National Rehabilitation Information Center (NRIC)
8455 Colesville Road, Suite 935
Silver Spring, MD 20910

NRIC provides information and referral services on disability and rehabilitation, including quick information and referral, and data base searches.

National Service Dog Center (NSDC)
289 Perimeter Road East
Renton, WA 98055-1329

NSDC, a program of Delta Society, assists people with disabilities to achieve greater independence and surmount barriers in their environment through the use of service dogs. NSDC provides advocacy on behalf of people with service dogs; education regarding service dog issues; information about the selection, training, stewardship, roles, and applications of service dogs; referral to service dog training programs and related resources; and research assistance.

National Temporal Bone Registry (NTBR)
Massachusetts Eye and Ear Infirmary
243 Charles Street
Boston, MA 02114-3096

NTBR is a nonprofit organization that coordinates the procurement of temporal bones upon the death of a donor, maintains a data base of all human temporal bone and associated brain tissue in the United States, and disseminates information to the public on temporal bone donation.

Registry of Interpreters for the Deaf, Inc. (RID)
8719 Colesville Road, Suite 310
Silver Spring, MD 20910

RID provides information about types of interpreting, evaluation, and certification of interpreters nationwide and maintains a list of certified interpreters.

Rehabilitation Engineering Research Center on Hearing Enhancement and Assistive Devices (RERC)
Lexington Center Inc.
30th Avenue and 75th Street
Jackson Heights, NY 11370

The RERC promotes and develops technological solutions to problems confronting individuals with hearing loss, and provides information and referral for consumer questions on assistive technology and research.

Rehabilitation Services Administration (RSA)
Office of Special Education and Rehabilitative Services
U.S. Department of Education
330 C Street S.W., Room 3228
Washington, D.C. 20202-2736

RSA promotes improved and expanded rehabilitation services for deaf and hard of hearing people and individuals with speech or language problems; provides technical assistance to RSA staff at state rehabilitation agencies, other public and private agencies, and individuals.

APPENDIX C

STATISTICS ON HEARING LOSS IN THE AGING POPULATION

More than 28 million Americans have a hearing loss; 80 percent of those affected have irreversible and permanent hearing damage.

More than one third of the United States population has a significant hearing loss by age 65.

Sixty percent of people with hearing loss are between the ages of 21 and 65.

Sensorineural damage (damage to the hair cells and cochlea caused by genetics or exposure to noise) is the largest, single form of hearing loss affecting 17 million Americans.

At least 15 percent of the United States population is affected by tinnitus.

Persons older than 50 years of age are twice as likely to have tinnitus.

Ménière's disease causes bilateral hearing loss in 5 to 20 percent of cases.

INDEX

Making the Most of Your Maturity With...

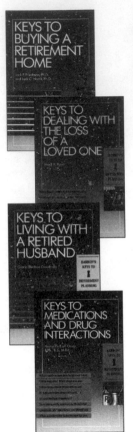

Barron's Keys to Retirement Planning
Each Key: Paperback: $5.95, Canada $7.95
Titles marked with asterisk * $6.95, Canada $8.95

Keys to...
Buying a Retirement Home
Friedman & Harris (0-8120-4476-2)
Choosing a Doctor
Lobanov & Shepard-Lobanov (0-8120-4621-8)
Dealing with the Loss of a Loved One
Kouri (0-8120-4676-5)
Fitness Over Fifty Murphy (0-8120-4514-9)
Living With a Retired Husband
Goodman (0-8120-4705-2)
*Living With Hearing Loss
Dugan (0-7641-0017-3)
Medications and Drug Interactions
Gever (0-8120-4749-4)
Menopause and Beyond Vierck (0-8120-4994-2)
Nutrition Over Fifty Murphy (0-8120-4512-2)
Planning for Long-term Custodial Care
Ness (0-8120-4593-9)
*Preparing a Will Jurinski (0-8120-4594-7)
Survival for Caregivers Kouri (0-8120-4814-8)
Understanding Alzheimer's Disease
Wolf-Klein & Levy (0-8120-4758-3)
Understanding Arthritis Vierck (0-8120-4731-1)
Understanding Medicare Gaffney (0-8120-4638-2)
Understanding Menopause and Beyond
Vierck (0-8120-4994-2)
Understanding Osteoporosis Rozek (0-8120-4664-1)
Understanding Social Security Benefits
Dickens & Crumbley (0-8120-4466-5)
Keys to Volunteering Vierck (0-8120-9507-3)

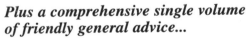

Plus a comprehensive single volume of friendly general advice...
Life Begins at 50:
A Handbook for Creative Retirement Planning
Leonard Hansen
Tips on retirement living, including handling your
money prudently, knowing about available health care,
Social Security and Medicare benefits, finding fun and
bargains in travel and entertainment. Paperback:
$12.95, Canada $16.95, 352 pp., (0-8120-4329-4)

Books may be purchased at your bookstore, or by mail from Barron's. Enclose check or money order for total amount plus sales tax where
applicable and add 15% for postage and handling (minimum charge $4.95). All books are paperback editions. Prices subject to change
without notice.
(#51) R 3/97

Barron's Educational Series, Inc.
250 Wireless Boulevard, Hauppauge, NY 11788
In Canada: Georgetown Book Warehouse • 34 Armstrong Avenue, Georgetown, Ont. L7G 4R9